# IMPROVING SERVICES FOR ASIAN DEAF CHILDREN

Parents' and professionals' perspectives

Rampaul Chamba, Waqar Ahmad and Lesley Jones

The POLICY
P~P
PRESS

First published in Great Britain in 1998 by

The Policy Press
University of Bristol
Rodney Lodge
Grange Road
Bristol BS8 4EA
UK

Tel    +44 (0)117 973 8797
Fax    +44 (0)117 973 7308
E-mail  tpp@bristol.ac.uk
Website http://www.bristol.ac.uk/Publications/TPP

ISBN 1 86134 129 6

**Rampaul Chamba** was a Research Fellow at the Ethnicity and Social Policy
Research Unit (ESPR), University of Bradford, during this project and is now a
doctoral student at the University of California, San Diego. **Waqar Ahmad** was
the Director of ESPR during this project, and is now the Professor of Primary
Care Research and Director, Centre for Research in Primary Care, Nuffield
Institute for Health, University of Leeds. **Lesley Jones** was a Senior Research
Fellow at ESPR while working on this project and is now at the Centre for
Research in Primary Care, University of Leeds. Lesley and Waqar are currently
working on an ESRC-funded study of Asian deaf young people.

Cover design by Qube Design Associates, Bristol.
Printed in Great Britain by Hobbs the Printers Ltd, Southampton.

# Contents

# Acknowledgements

This research project would not have been possible without the support of a number of individuals and agencies. The Department of Health (DoH), through its Ethnic Minority Health Access programme, provided generous funding for the project. We thank Miss Veena Bahl, the Departmental Adviser, Ethnic Minority Health and the DoH for financial support. Equally, we are grateful to the many parents and professionals whose accounts form the basis of this report.

A number of other people helped at different stages. We thank Gill Parry, Gulshan Karbani, Kulvir Lal, Mushtaq Mir, Nuzhat Khan and Liz Kernohan for helpful discussions. Aliya Darr conducted some of the interviews. Gohar Nisar, our Deaf consultant on a related project, offered guidance at various points. Allison Campbell provided excellent secretarial support as well as occasional counselling.

The project began its life at the Social Policy Research Unit, University of York, where we received moral and intellectual support from Sally Baldwin and Hazel Qureshi and administrative help from Jenny Bowes, Sally Pulleyn and Teresa Anderson. We thank them all for their help.

It is a pleasure also to acknowledge the support of our advisory committee consisting of Vinod Kumar (National Children's Society), Jonathan Phillips (Social Services Inspectorate), Bob Mueller (St James' Hospital, Leeds), Liz Kernohan (Bradford Health), Melissa James (National Deaf Children's Society), Nuzhat Khan (Bradford Social Services), Jill Jones (Rotherham Social Services), Susan Gregory (University of Birmingham), Sandra Smith (independent researcher) and Ali Iftikhar Raja (visiting student from Pakistan). Vinod and Jonathan chaired the committee at different times. Jonathan, Susan and Melissa also provided much valued feedback on earlier drafts; in particular, Jonathan and Susan helped make the recommendations much clearer.

# Executive summary

## Introduction

Little research attention has been paid to minority ethnic deaf children, although the need for improved service provision for minority ethnic deaf adults has been acknowledged in some studies.

Recognising this gap, the DoH commissioned research on services for Asian deaf pre-school age children.

## The study

This qualitative study focused on parental and professional perspectives on improving health and social care for deaf children. The project aimed to provide a fuller understanding of parents' perceptions and their experiences of children's deafness, their interaction with health, education and social services and types of support they found helpful. It also aimed to provide practitioners' perspectives on service delivery and means of improving services; and to assess how health commissioners established priorities and mechanisms for purchasing and monitoring services for deaf children.

Interviews were undertaken with parents and professionals in West Yorkshire. The final sample included 70 respondents. Twenty-six interviews were conducted with parents: 21 with mothers and five with fathers. Parents with deaf children (upper half of moderate to profound) aged five or under were selected for interview. They were interviewed in the language of their choice, and, if requested, by a researcher of the same gender. Three children had multiple disabilities. Of the 44 practitioners: 18 were health service providers, 14 were peripatetic teachers, six were social services staff and six were health commissioners.

## Findings

### Policy framework and commissioning services

Recent policy legislation, including the 1989 Children Act, 1990 NHS and Community Care Act, 1993 Education Act and 1995 Carers Act, demands a reorganisation of services provided to disabled children and their families. This legislation provides scope for improving services for disabled children and their carers in response to their assessed needs and preferences. It also encourages innovation and interagency collaboration between statutory agencies, as well as with the voluntary sector.

Overall, local demographic characteristics and epidemiology of deafness played little role in purchasing services and agreeing budgets. The presumed higher prevalence of childhood deafness among the Asian community was not reflected in enhanced budgets for services for deaf children. Purchasers felt needs assessment and demographic profiling were of limited help in identifying specific needs, and purchasing mechanisms worked at too broad a level to allow close monitoring or evaluation. Priority setting was a politically fraught activity and ethnicity did not have a high status in considerations about budgets. When ethnic sensitivity is specified in contracts, it is at a broad level and detail is worked out by the trust. Monitoring data provided by trusts are about activity and costs, not about quality and sensitivity. The ability of purchasers to effect change was thus limited, and change, some argued, depended on medium to long-term planning and individual commitment within organisations.

## Screening and diagnosis

The lack of nationally-agreed protocols for neonatal screening has led to different policies across health districts. Universal screening was not seen to be cost-effective. Professionals felt technical as well as other problems (population inflow) meant that no screening programme could be effective in identifying all deaf children. Some of the areas had 'at-risk' registers to help identify families with a history of deafness, which facilitated earlier diagnosis. At-risk screening also lacked standard protocols. Practitioners felt that the combination of the at-risk register, distraction tests and parental vigilance ensured that the majority of deaf children were identified. This was seen to work for Asian as well as other deaf children. However, this emphasis on 'high-risk' screening led to fears that 'low-risk' children may not be identified sufficiently quickly. In terms of improving screening coverage, it was felt that considerable improvements could be made by using existing screening systems more effectively rather than introducing additional tests.

Purchasers and providers felt distraction tests to be a vital part of the service. Key limitations included conducting tests in rooms without sound proofing, often in the presence of siblings; health visitors not having knowledge of the child's home language to help assess speech development; professionals' low expectations of Asian and other disadvantaged children in terms of language development; and training requirements of health visitors. Health visitors were valued by parents although some parents criticised them and other professionals for not taking parental concerns seriously. Parents were critical that distraction tests sometimes failed to identify deafness leading to delays in diagnosis and necessary support. Parents had little contact with general practitioners (GPs) and felt that GPs were poorly informed about deafness.

There were different views on whether Asian children are being diagnosed later than white children. Most practitioners felt at-risk registers and improved service coordination had led to earlier diagnosis as shown by the reduced age of fitting hearing aids. Other practitioners felt Asian children may be being diagnosed later than white children. Missed appointments, visits to the sub-continent, failure of distraction tests, language barriers and not taking parents' concerns seriously were suggested as reasons. Parents were sympathetic to problems of reaching diagnosis quickly but had concerns about the negative impact of late diagnosis on their child's development.

## Access and communication

*Improving the appointments system:* many professionals, mainly consultants, felt attendance at appointments was poor due to: visits abroad; lack of parental concern about children; perceived parental bias in favour of boys than girls when attending appointments; and presumed unreasonable expectations of external help such as for transport. These reasons were contested by parents and by some professionals. Parents' concerns included: long delays before and between appointments; unhelpful receptionists; delays in seeing professionals even with a specific appointment time; too short a time with the professional during consultation; inflexibility of appointments which did not take account of childcare or work commitments; lack of interpreting support; difficulty of juggling appointments between different clinics and different provider trusts; and appointments being changed at short notice. Some of these problems result from the block booking system and could be solved by better administration, and improved communication between professionals and between professionals and parents.

*Disclosure of diagnosis:* appropriate disclosure is vital for parents' understanding and acceptance of deafness. On the whole, parents were satisfied with disclosure. Disclosures which were sympathetic, sensitive, unhurried, and offered opportunities to ask questions were valued. Some peripatetic teachers felt the diagnosis was poorly explained and the setting (often no private room to talk to parents) was not conducive to sensitive handling of parents' concerns and information needs. There was a lack of clarity between the roles of the consultant and the peripatetic teacher. Some parents felt the consultant should offer fuller explanations while others felt this was best done by the peripatetic teacher. Some social workers of the deaf felt that there was a clear role for them in providing emotional support to parents. This was impeded by a lack of clarity in professional division of labour and poor interagency collaboration.

*Information:* parents wanted better information on causation and the implications of deafness for language development and felt consultants should encourage parents to return to ask further questions. Mostly, parents relied more on peripatetic teachers for such information. Professionals felt Asian families remained poorly served in terms of information. Language barriers, poor interpreting facilities, shortage of bilingual staff and limited translated materials contributed to an information vacuum. Consequently, Asian parents coped and made decisions with more limited information and fewer resources than white parents. This is more problematic for Asian mothers as more of them have difficulty in using English.

*Causation:* few parents had a clear idea of causation, suggesting a need for fuller explanation of the child's deafness. Professionals held differing views on the utility of genetic counselling. There was no system for routine referral of 'at-risk' families for genetic counselling and no professional had explicit responsibility for referral. Many parents are being denied access to genetic knowledge and information which they may find useful.

*Interpreting:* using spouses, family or friends as interpreters was taken for granted by parents, and by some professionals. Poor interpreting services and problems of communication caused major concerns to practitioners as well as purchasers. No locality had a dedicated interpreting service; most health visitors and peripatetic teachers relied on overstretched hospital-wide services with interpreters who did not have expert knowledge of deafness; obtaining interpreting support could be slow and lack of training of interpreters and of professionals in using interpreters is of concern.

## Amplification support

*Hearing aids:* on the whole, parents were satisfied with hearing aids although their views often differed from professionals. Many parents felt their experience of care of the deaf child meant they knew more than professionals about how and when to use aids. Parents and professionals differed about the regular use of hearing aids. Parents and children required time to adjust to using aids. This was influenced by the obtrusiveness of the hearing aid, especially for very young children and potential stigma and victimisation in schools. Some practitioners felt the increased prevalence of deafness among the Asian population should be taken into account in setting budgets for amplification support. The service was felt to be under-resourced although it may be seen to have an appropriate allocation if seen simply in terms of population size. Lack of clear division in the budgets, between support for children and adults, was problematic and policies on commercial hearing aids differed between authorities. Provision of aids was not well integrated between health services and education services in some of the localities.

*Cochlear implants:* parents were either against implants or remained ambivalent. Consultants and peripatetic teachers were the main source of information. Parents remained unconvinced about the effectiveness of implants; some knew of cases where they felt implants improved hearing too little to justify the discomfort, and potential 'permanent damage' caused by the procedure. Practitioners were divided about cochlear implants with healthcare staff being more positive than teachers. Teachers felt that some parents were being pressured into accepting implants; some consultants were puzzled by parental hostility or ambivalence towards a potential 'cure' for the child's deafness.

## Language, communication and education

*British Sign Language (BSL) and spoken languages:* teachers were divided in their opinions about the relationship between BSL and spoken languages such as Punjabi/Urdu and English. Some regarded BSL as a separate language; some saw a relationship between spoken English and sign-supported English; others argued that BSL had greater resemblance to the grammatical structure of Punjabi/Urdu. Teachers were also divided in advice they gave to parents about children's language development. Denial of access to mother tongue to the previous generation of deaf Asian children was regarded by some teachers as racist; others still favoured only spoken English, in addition to BSL, and felt that learning more than one spoken language causes confusion for the child. Those who supported multilingualism (sign language, English plus home language) emphasised the importance of the deaf child developing a positive cultural identity.

*Communication strategies:* parental communication strategies were influenced by teachers' advice, previous experiences, linguistic preferences and concerns about education and integration in the deaf and/or ethnic community. All parents showed support for spoken language development but used a variety of languages with children including home language. Some remained confused about language choice complicated by uncertainty about the degree of the child's deafness. Advice from some professionals to only use English with deaf children was seen as undermining the child's cultural identity and compromising communication with the wider family. Many mothers were learning BSL or sign-supported English but few fathers made an effort to learn sign language.

*Schooling:* parental decisions about schooling were informed by the child's characteristics, including the degree of deafness, parents' personal preferences and appropriate resources in schools. Parents saw costs and benefits of both mainstream schools and schools for deaf children. Some were pleasantly surprised by the educational achievements of children at schools for deaf children. Parents remained concerned about the relative lack of emphasis on religious and cultural identity in deaf children's education but welcomed initiatives to do this in some schools.

*Speech and language therapy:* none of the children were as yet receiving speech and language therapy. However, the need to provide speech therapy in the children's home languages was noted by some parents and professionals.

### Family life and support

Much of the daily caring of the deaf child was done by parents, largely mothers. The wider family provided valued emotional and practical support for many parents. This support varied widely and depended on the history of deafness within the family, household composition and the geographical proximity of family members. Not all parents of deaf children felt that they had the level of support that they would have liked or found it helpful when provided.

Families with a previous history of deafness found it easier to understand and accept the diagnosis. Their experience of deafness also helped in earlier diagnosis and in establishing support for the child.

## Collaboration and service coordination

*Health services:* problems of coordination hampered collaborative work between professionals within the same agencies, as well as between agencies. Often services were split between hospitals within the same provider trust leading to duplication and confusion for parents who may be requested to attend different hospitals for different procedures or for different children. Communication remained poor between health visitors and secondary care; health visitors felt they could be more effective if they were routinely informed about children's progress through the system. GPs remained marginal to services for deaf children. Parents found the boundaries between different agencies puzzling and unhelpful. They found it difficult to compartmentalise issues of caring, language choice and development, housing, resources, equipment and costs to fit the remit of particular agencies. Access to sign language teaching and information on deafness and deaf culture was facilitated largely by teachers, who often assumed the role of 'key worker'.

*Social services:* social services had little contact with parents of deaf children. Social services may have a role in the emotional support of parents as well as provision of support and guidance about aids and benefits. The involvement of social services remained marginal in all study sites.

*Voluntary organisations:* parents made little use of voluntary organisations, although they had information about these from peripatetic teachers. Most parents knew about such help but found access to support groups difficult or unnecessary; parents rated health and education services more relevant than the voluntary sector.

*Interagency working:* good working arrangements between health and peripatetic education services in some areas were encouraging and offer possibilities for other localities. We found no examples of a similar level or quality of interagency working between health and social services, or between health and the voluntary sector.

# ONE

# Introduction

Although there is considerable research literature on ethnicity, health and healthcare (eg, Ahmad, 1993; Smaje, 1994; Ahmad and Atkin, 1996b), there is little research on minority ethnic children (Kurtz, 1993). The limited literature focusing on children is concentrated in areas such as haemoglobinopathies, nutritional disorders, learning disability and infant mortality (Anionwu, 1993; Parsons et al, 1993; Kurtz, 1993; Ahmad and Atkin, 1996a).

For ethnic minorities, little attention has been devoted to disability and chronic illness, especially as they affect children. The scant and, in terms of quality, highly variable literature on ethnicity and deafness has concentrated on adults and there remains a lack of research on minority ethnic deaf children (Sharma and Love, 1991; Badat and Whall-Roberts, 1994; Ahmad et al, 1998; Ahmad et al, forthcoming). The need for improved service provision for minority ethnic deaf people is highlighted in recent publications (eg, Ahmad et al, 1998; Ahmad et al, forthcoming; Chamba et al, 1998). As Ahmad et al (1998) note, a range of initiatives have developed around ethnicity and deafness in recent years but a variety of problems remain (see also Darr et al, 1997):

- there are problems of access to services; spoken and sign language support is not always available and families often have to make decisions on the basis of inadequate or incomplete information;
- minority ethnic deaf people do not have adequate representation in Deaf[1] organisations, and many experience racism from within the Deaf community;
- provision in statutory agencies is often made through the 'specialist worker' approach which puts unacceptable burdens on the minority ethnic workers and often leads to the employing agency 'dumping' all minority ethnic cases onto that worker;
- young deaf people and their parents were concerned that earlier education policies had encouraged them to use only English as a spoken language at the expense of other spoken (home) languages; this had led to many young people having little communication with those family members who did not use British Sign Language

(BSL) or spoken English and deaf people had only limited knowledge of their ethnic and religious background;
• services were poorly coordinated both within and between agencies, thus exacerbating problems of access.

Recognising this gap in available research, this project focuses on services for Asian deaf children under five years of age. Estimates suggest that deafness is more prevalent among sections of the Asian community than in the white population but findings are inconsistent across localities (Ahmad et al, 1998, ch 3). Very little of the literature on minority ethnic deaf children focuses on parental experiences; the only piece of research in this area we are aware of is a Masters level dissertation (Meherali, 1985 and more recent work by Mahon et al, 1995). To our knowledge no research has been conducted which focuses both on Asian parents' and professionals' perspectives in relation to general service provision issues, including the process of diagnosis. The aims of the research reported here were to provide:
• a fuller understanding of parents' perceptions and experiences of their child's deafness;
• the parents' and service providers' perspectives on the nature of service delivery and, especially, the means of improving services.

The research is based on detailed interviews with 26 parents of pre-school deaf children and 44 professionals from health, education and social services. The study was conducted in West Yorkshire. Details of the methods are given in Appendix A. Appendix B provides brief profiles of families interviewed for this research.

## Structure of the book

An executive summary, highlighting the significant findings precedes this introduction. Following this introduction, the research findings are presented in six substantive chapters. The final chapter makes detailed recommendations for improving services.

Chapter 2 charts the parental journey to seek an understanding of and support for their child's condition, from initial suspicion to obtaining the diagnosis of deafness. Chapter 3 explores the nature and quality of support from different professionals once the child has been diagnosed as deaf. The social impact of deafness on parents and the wider family is important to explore, and is the subject of Chapter 4.

In Chapters 5 and 6, the focus is on professionals. Chapter 5 discusses a number of important aspects in screening for and diagnosing deafness. Thus, it focuses on interagency and interprofessional collaboration and coordination of services, the role of distraction tests and other means of screening for deafness, and professionals' ideas about aetiology. In Chapter 6, we explore professionals' perspectives on improving services.

Chapter 7 integrates the accounts of parents and professionals in a brief synthesis of the main findings and puts these in broader policy and practice framework. Finally, detailed recommendations for services are given in Chapter 8. As this research was supported by the Department of Health (DoH), the recommendations are targeted at the health services. However, the study has important implications for social services, education and the voluntary sector and many of the general recommendations would apply equally across agencies.

## Note

[1] We follow the convention of using 'deaf' to denote people with deafness as a generic term, and 'Deaf' to refer to those who use BSL as the means of communication and regard themselves as a linguistic minority.

# TWO

# Negotiating diagnosis: initial suspicions and contact with services

This chapter charts the journey from initial concerns about the child's hearing to the diagnosis of deafness. We describe parents' initial suspicions and contact with professionals such as health visitors, general practitioners (GPs), and others. Disclosure of diagnosis, information given during the diagnostic consultation, and parents' reactions to diagnosis are discussed. Teachers of the deaf often work closely with health professionals; we explore their role in the diagnostic process and in supporting parents. Finally, we explore parental concerns about the speed with which diagnosis was made and their views about causation.

## Initial suspicions

Concern about the child's development may be raised by parents, other family members, or by health visitors or other professionals. A family history of deafness may make parents and health professionals vigilant about the child's hearing. The first part of this chapter discusses parents' initial suspicions and their experiences with health professionals.

### Initial concerns

There is considerable variability in parental concerns about a child and initial contact with practitioners. Parents are usually the first to suspect potential hearing loss or speech delay. Where parents had a family history of deafness, their own and professionals' vigilance led to earlier diagnosis. With no prior history of deafness, diagnosis could take longer and parental suspicion was often deflected by minor illnesses or assumptions about the child's 'stubbornness'.

Concern often arose when children's communication skills fell below those of other children of a similar age. In a few cases, deafness was related to meningitis or existed in addition to other disabilities. In some instances, parents found out about hearing loss through routine developmental tests.

Where parents were concerned about a child's hearing, they consulted GPs or health visitors, often leading to referral for hearing assessment. However, action which followed was often slow. For example, one child who was regarded as 'slow' but who could speak a few words was referred to health professionals; his hearing tests began at the age of six months. He was finally diagnosed as having a hearing impairment when he was four. Equally, there were children who were not identified through routine testing and about whose hearing parents had few concerns. In one child's case, it was nursery school teachers who alerted the parents and professionals to suspected hearing loss.

### The health visitor's role

A recurrent question asked by parents was why the hearing loss was not identified at the distraction test conducted at the age of six to eight months. In some cases, parents knew that the onset of hearing impairment is highly variable and may arise at different times; or because of differences in children's communication abilities, hearing loss can be difficult to identify. More often, however, parents were bemused by this problem and found it difficult to understand the subsequent onset of hearing loss, or the problem in reaching diagnosis. For some, this was related to 'not being heard' by professionals, the apparent carelessness of professionals, and fears that delay in diagnosis was deleterious to speech and sign language development.

Parents who were unhappy about distraction tests felt that the health visitors should have identified deafness earlier and made appropriate referral. The subsequent diagnosis also led to parental concerns about aetiology: when, if not present at the time of the distraction test, did hearing loss take place? Parents' views on causation are discussed later.

Some parents' accounts suggest that guidelines for hearing assessment are not always followed. The experience of a parent described earlier, whose child was diagnosed at the age of four, stated that the distraction test was conducted three or four times. The guidelines are that these tests should not be conducted more than twice, following which a referral should be made if hearing loss is suspected. Elsewhere, a parent had doubts about her child's hearing but the child nevertheless 'passed' the test.

Not all parents had negative experiences with health visitors, although there was an appeal from many for health visitors (and other professionals) to take parents' concerns more seriously. Some parents were complimentary about the support they received from health visitors, or felt that they were 'doing enough'. Parental concerns about the child would clearly be expected to be broader than the immediate issue of deafness. The provision of more general support and advice from health visitors was important to parents and much appreciated.

More critically, concern was raised about the precise role of the health visitors. Parents noted, for example, that the health visitors' contact with the parent and child lasted for a relatively short time and that a longer-term commitment would be welcomed. Once the health visitor had made a referral, parents felt their involvement had diminished and remained limited even after the formal diagnosis. More broadly, some felt that health visitors should act as 'key workers' and facilitate the coordination of support services.

## General practitioners

Similar reservations to those noted above were expressed about GPs. Important features of parents' experiences were the GPs' relatively minor involvement in identifying hearing loss, and their limited reliance on GPs for specialist advice. To some parents, this mattered little as referral or contact with the hearing centre or hospital had already been made through the health visitor. Most contact with GPs was for minor ailments and other routine consultations. In these cases, GPs were found to be generally helpful. However, some parents felt that their support needs would be better met if the GPs played a more active role in relation to their child's deafness.

Concern about GPs' lack of knowledge about deafness did not appear frequently but some parents felt that this compromised the GPs' ability to help. Some parents would have valued such contact with a sympathetic and knowledgeable GP, especially between lengthy waits between appointments at the hospital. Parents also felt that GPs do not always take parents' concerns seriously and have limited ability to communicate with deaf children.

## Appointment system

Hospital and clinic appointments play a crucial role in mediating interaction between practitioners and parents. Problems in this area are likely to compromise the quality of interaction between professionals and parents, and contribute to delays in diagnosis and care of the deaf child. An understanding of parents' concerns about appointments will also contextualise some criticisms raised by practitioners (discussed in Chapters 5 and 6).

It is important to acknowledge that some parents found appointments satisfactory. Flexibility, empathy and perceived professional competence were particularly valued. However, a number of problems were identified, including:

- lengthy lead-in period for appointments;
- letters of appointment not being clear;
- administrative incompetence on the part of hospital staff;
- poor communication between specialists and primary care;
- lengthy waiting times despite having a specific time for an appointment;
- perceived inflexibility of receptionists who did not allow parents to rearrange appointments at more convenient times;
- very limited time spent in actual consultation.

Parents also perceived a lack of sympathy on the part of professionals with the difficulty they had in keeping appointments. Demands of paid employment posed particular problems. For example, one father reduced his working hours and changed his shifts to ensure that he could attend appointments.

Another source of difficulty stemmed from keeping track of appointments when parents had more than one deaf child, often reinforced by not having appropriate or readily available transport. For some, this was exacerbated by different children having appointments in different hospitals for reasons unknown to parents.

## Diagnosing deafness

Here, we describe parents' contact with practitioners including: communication with practitioners; quality and quantity of information; disclosing diagnosis; reaction to diagnosis; and speed with which deafness was identified.

### Communication with practitioners

Parents of deaf children come into contact with a wide range of professionals, including senior clinical medical officers, community paediatricians, consultant ENT (ear, nose and throat) surgeons, educational audiologists, audiological physicians, audiological scientists, and paediatric audiological technicians in addition to health visitors and GPs. While a structure guides and informs parents' contact with these professionals, processes of referral undergo adjustments to take account of individual children's characteristics, and local service organisation. We describe broad concerns before considering specific issues.

One important concern related to the short duration of consultations. It was felt that consultations were too brief and more time was needed to explain what was wrong and to give parents the opportunity to ask questions. The demands on consultants were well understood but parents felt that more could be done to make consultations satisfactory, including having other staff to ease the consultant's load. Sufficient time was perceived to be particularly important in the first appointment.

The limited time spent with parents is not conducive to exchanging information and parents expressed concern about lack of information given, such as on implications of the hearing loss for speech and language development. Parents noted a variety of problems regarding information, without there being a clear consensus. Some were happy with the tests but not with the quality or range of information; others felt they did not have sufficient time to digest the written information provided; others valued the opportunity to speak to practitioners directly and felt that this was not always possible. The last was favoured particularly in that it allowed parents to check their understandings with the practitioners. Positively, one parent, reflecting on her experience of contact with services over a longer time-span, had noted positive changes in doctors' ability and willingness to explain diagnosis or procedures and inform parents about options and services. Her experiences with an older deaf child, about 10 years earlier, were particularly negative.

Interpreting support was usually provided when requested, but was not available at all times. Some parents were content to use their partners or family members for interpretation. The lack of interpreting support did not attract much comment, although one father resented having to take time off work to take the child to the local school for the deaf because staff had difficulty in communicating with his wife who could not speak English.

## The diagnostic consultation

The diagnostic consultation, when parents are told about the formal diagnosis, is an important event. Here we consider: disclosure; parents' reaction to the diagnosis; and contact after the diagnosis. These three phases appear to be pivotal to the diagnostic process. Respectively, they relate, first, to the manner in which potentially upsetting information about diagnosis and prognosis is conveyed by the practitioner, usually a consultant. Secondly, parental reaction to the diagnosis is and can be varied and needs discussion. Thirdly, while all parents' reaction to the formal diagnosis was of shock and grief, parents varied in their desire, willingness and ability to ask questions and seek information about the implications of hearing loss for their child's development.

*Disclosure:* on the whole, parents felt that diagnoses were disclosed in a sympathetic and professional way. Where there were criticisms by some parents, these related to the 'unsympathetic' manner of the consultant and a perceived lack of consideration that the diagnosis may be traumatic for parents. The shortness of the consultation only made this perception worse.

For example, parents of one child, who did not feel that their child's hearing was appropriately investigated, were dissatisfied with the matter of fact way in which they were told about the child's deafness. They felt that the diagnosis should have been disclosed sympathetically and that other parents may not be as confident as themselves in objecting to unsympathetic and mechanistic disclosure.

*Parents' reaction to the diagnosis:* parents' reactions to diagnoses were varied. Nearly all parents stated that their reaction was one of grief or shock, often accompanied by disbelief or denial. In time, feelings of grief and shock were tempered by meeting other deaf children and finding comfort in the acknowledgement that it is 'Allah who gives' such tests as well as the courage and capacity to cope with adversity. Parents talked of their 'minds being in turmoil' at being given the diagnosis and considering it 'the worst thing' that could have happened to them.

Anger, disbelief and denial often existed alongside feelings of upset and shock. One parent, for example, while angry that the doctors should suggest the child is deaf, was at the same time grateful that the problem had been identified early. Disbelief was also expressed as 'why me', so commonly used by people in such circumstances as well as feeling, on the part of some parents, that some wrong doing had precipitated deafness. At times, parents believed that the diagnosis was based on inaccurate testing as it seemed inconsistent with their own assessment of the child's speech.

However, many recognised the inherent difficulty of making definitive statements about a child's hearing. Others recognised that they were in denial, while, with hindsight, the evidence for the child being deaf was clear. Some only accepted the diagnosis following a second opinion, in one case privately paid for.

*Communication with practitioners:* for parents, flexibility, sensitivity, empathy with parents' circumstances and needs, and sympathy were important practitioner attributes. Parents' responses suggest considerable variation in the opportunities for questions and in their own desire for information. Time is required for parents to think of information needs or absorb given information. Further, as noted, many parents were in a state of grief or emotional turmoil which did not facilitate well-considered exchange with professionals about information needs or prognosis.

One way of improving communication is by involving other practitioners during the consultation or at a later date. As such, in some areas it has become standard practice for teachers of deaf children to be present at the diagnostic consultation or to contact parents shortly after the diagnosis. In some areas, teachers played an important role in explaining, among other things, the implications of the child's hearing loss and act as a key resource for parents. However, some parents would still have welcomed more time and opportunity for discussion with the consultant during the diagnostic consultation.

Lack of explanation for the deafness, prognosis, language development, prospects for a 'cure' or a 'normal life' troubled many parents and some felt that they, at best, had only partial understandings of these issues. Written information only went so far; having someone to talk to allowed parents to check out their own understandings, seek clarifications and acquire information which was timely, related to concrete issues as they arose, rather than given in the abstract. The teachers performed this role for many parents.

*Information from health and education practitioners:* as noted, the division of labour between health and education practitioners means that, following diagnosis, only a limited amount of time is spent with parents by consultants or audiologists. Instead the coordinating and information-giving role is fulfilled primarily by teachers of deaf children.

On the whole, parents valued the opportunity to gain relevant information during the diagnostic consultation although, as discussed above, they varied both in the kind of information they wanted and the way it should be provided. This related also to information from paediatric audiological technicians about hearing aids, batteries and cochlear implants. Referring to the diagnostic consultation, very few parents mentioned that they were given any information about the implications of the child's hearing loss for speech and language development; who they should see next, such as a genetic counsellor or teacher; or information about the outcome of an operation. Usually, this information came from the teacher in later meetings. All parents were complementary of the role of teachers.

The content of this information, and the preferred method varied between parents. There was a desire for more information in audio or visual (video and picture) form or, more importantly, in a form appropriate to the individual parents' needs. Some expressed a need for more translated information, including information on cochlear implants.

For those parents who still disagreed with the diagnosis, the information about tests and their results appeared inadequate or unsatisfactory. In these cases, more time and work was needed for an informed understanding. Some found diagnostic classifications such as 'profound' or 'moderate' deafness or references to frequency bands confusing. More meaningful information informing parents of the child's current needs and future development was appreciated. Those parents who had a child with other disabilities as well as deafness needed additional information, particularly where they felt that the deafness was less problematic than, what for them, was the more serious condition.

The role of information in keeping parents informed about their child's deafness and the developmental process is important. It also helps to reduce, among other things, the sense of isolation and helplessness felt by some parents in coming to terms with their child's deafness. In principle, all members of the multidisciplinary team involved in the welfare of a deaf child have a responsibility to ensure that parents' concerns and questions are addressed, but it is clear that some parents felt that they had not received adequate information and support.

*The speed of diagnosis:* here we describe parents' views about the speed with which deafness was diagnosed. Early identification of hearing loss is crucial for linguistic and intellectual development and there are guidelines in paediatric audiology to facilitate referral and early diagnosis. While these guidelines outline how referral and procedures should unfold, operationalisation of these guidelines to assess the quality and efficiency of audiological services is much more problematic. A range of individual factors, including non-attendance by families, other disabilities in the case of children leaving neonatal intensive care units and the need for surgical interventions may contribute to how referral procedures unfold. The mean age of detection and hearing aid fitting are seen to represent some of the key points to judge the quality and efficacy of care.

In interviews, parents were asked to recall time lapses between appointments and the process of referral and their feelings about and reasons for perceived delayed diagnosis. Not all parents were able to give detailed accounts of the process of referral or delays between various stages of the diagnostic process. However, parents did express views about the overall speed with which referral and testing took place. Some were dissatisfied with the speed with which their child's hearing loss was detected but this was not universal. For those parents who felt that diagnoses should have been made earlier, there may be sound medical or other reasons why this was not possible. It is not clear from parents' accounts whether the perceived delay can be attributed to a single factor, such as the failure of the distraction test to identify hearing loss or delays in the appointments system. Rather, different parents experienced problems at different phases of their contact with practitioners.

Parents who already had older deaf children were pleased that they managed to have deafness diagnosed quickly in their younger children. This may be due to parents' greater experience in identifying clues and/or or heightened vigilance on the part of professionals. Even where diagnosis took considerable time, parents were often understanding of the potential problems in reaching diagnosis. For one parent, although an earlier diagnosis would have been desirable – her child was not diagnosed until the age of six years – she felt it was unfair to blame practitioners who had routinely tested the child.

In some cases, there was a more explicit attribution of blame to health practitioners. For example, one parent blamed the health visitor, GP and local health clinic for not finding out about her child's deafness earlier, although she had not discussed these concerns with the relevant practitioners. This mother felt that her concerns were not taken seriously by professionals – a criticism also made by other parents.

## Information about causation

Views on causation featured frequently in parents' accounts. Not knowing the cause of deafness was a source of anxiety. This concern was compounded by uncertainty about the time or age at which hearing loss arose. Due to insufficient clinical information at the time of the diagnosis, health practitioners were often unclear about the precise aetiology of hearing loss. Nevertheless, the views expressed by parents suggest that health practitioners should devote more time to addressing concerns around aetiology, even when such knowledge may be limited.

Parents were given a wide range of possible reasons for their child's deafness. These included nerve damage, asphyxiation during birth, neuro-deafness, or hereditary causes.

Parents' understandings of causation differed widely. Some felt that no explanation had been given, or practitioners did not know themselves. A number of parents had no knowledge of causation and wanted to know more about this. The type of information parents wanted included:

- Was the child deaf at birth?
- If not, at what point might deafness have occurred?
- Could it have been diagnosed earlier?
- Why was it, for example, that their child of six became deaf?
- Why was there a perceived high prevalence of deafness among Asian people?

Also, parents wanted information which was clear and easily understandable rather than vague, cryptic or technical.

With the exception of two families, all of the parents interviewed in this study were of Pakistani Muslim origin. Consanguinity featured frequently in Muslim parents' understandings of causation. This either stemmed from information given to parents by practitioners, personal understandings about inheritance and family history of deafness where it existed, or from other sources.

For some parents, although the genetic basis for deafness was possible, they did not discount other potential causes. Nor did a family history of deafness make the genetic explanation straightforward to understand. Ideas about inheritance and marriage with close kin did not feature as the sole explanation but often coexisted with other factors such as illness and medical complications.

Not all parents agreed with the consanguinity explanation. Where consanguinity was given as the principal reason for deafness some objections were expressed by parents who felt this to be an attack by health professionals on cherished cultural practices.

Views about genetic counselling varied considerably. Some parents had contact with genetic services to establish the likelihood of deafness in future children. Others did not want contact until they knew what caused their child's deafness or did not believe genetic counselling could help. Other parents had decided not to have any more children and felt counselling had nothing to offer them. There were also some reservations about the credibility of genetic counselling. One mother, for example, described the situation of a friend who was told that there was a strong chance of her future children being deaf; they had two more children, both hearing.

## Summary

Parental vigilance alongside routine testing facilitated the identification of deafness in most children. Parents were generally satisfied with communication and access, although some problems were highlighted. These related to problems with the appointments system, short duration of consultations and perceived unsympathetic attitude of some consultants and receptionists. Teachers of the deaf played a key role in information-giving and service coordination.

Parental reactions to diagnosis included feelings of grief and loss mixed with anger and denial. However, for some, these emotions were coupled with relief that the deafness had been identified and support could be established. Parents were generally happy with the speed of diagnosis, although some felt that their concerns were not taken sufficiently seriously by practitioners. Previous family history of deafness often led to speedier diagnosis. Parents' views on causation varied. Many were poorly informed about causation, often having a vague idea of deafness being related to consanguinity, an attribution many parents questioned and resented. Chapter 3 considers parental interaction with services following the diagnosis.

# THREE

# After the diagnosis: adjustment and interaction with services

The diagnosis of deafness may represent a pivotal point for parents in their contact with health and other services, but service contact continues to be important after the diagnosis. In addition to having to come to terms with having a deaf child, parents have to start planning for the future, including amplification support and contact with educational or peripatetic support services. Following diagnosis, the peripatetic support services, specifically teachers, play an important role in supporting both parents and deaf children, providing information about services and technical aids, and informing about developmental needs.

This chapter focuses on a number of inter-related issues which parents confront after diagnosis. Following diagnosis, parents often need to continue contact with audiological services for hearing aids or surgical procedures, including cochlear implants. We discuss parents' perceptions of amplification support and their child's needs. Contact with the peripatetic support service plays an important part in continuing amplification support and facilitating sign language, and speech and language therapy. We describe parents' views of their child's language and communication development and about communicating with the child. In addition to ongoing support from health and education services and the immediate family, support is available from other organisations. We explore parents' experiences of other support services and their satisfaction with the information and help provided. Finally, we discuss some areas of unmet need and the kind of interventions parents find helpful.

## Amplification support for the deaf child

Following diagnosis, contact with health and the peripatetic education service is concerned with the support needs of the deaf child. Both practitioners and parents are faced with important decisions concerning the best support for the child. Practitioners need to advise on the appropriateness of hearing aids and radio aids, consider cochlear implants and sometimes perform surgery to treat conductive loss. Parents need to understand the nature of their child's deafness, developmental changes and various forms of support such as hearing aids and cochlear implants, and decide the best course of action. As discussed below, parents' decisions are made in the context of perceived short- and long-term implications of these medical interventions for their deaf child. These decisions are also informed by parents' preferences about, for example, speech or sign language, and if speech, then the choice of spoken language(s). This section will consider parents' views about hearing aids and cochlear implants, respectively.

## Hearing aids

The diversity of responses and views about hearing aids and cochlear implants suggests considerable ambivalence and anxiety. Several parents did not comment explicitly on hearing aids either because their child had not received one yet, or they were perceived to be unproblematic.

Some parents were satisfied with the information and explanations they had been given by the paediatric audiological technicians and other professionals about hearing aids and batteries; others were more ambivalent, reflecting a wider ambivalence with the whole issue of their child's deafness. For example, one mother was satisfied with the child's hearing aid, but did not necessarily regard it as the solution: she was still hoping for a procedure which would give her child hearing.

Satisfaction with hearing aids also appeared to extend to the speed with which hearing aids were fitted, though this was not universal. For some parents, the delay in obtaining a hearing aid was unjustifiably long, a concern also shared by the teachers. The main issues raised by parents related to difficulties with the child's use of the hearing aids. In some cases, the child did not like wearing the aid, a problem which was further complicated by some children having ear infections and coughs and colds. However, some parents felt that the smaller post-aural aids were easier to adjust to, especially for very young children. Parents also preferred these aids as they were less conspicuous – some talked about being distressed at the prospect of people staring at their children if they were wearing aids which made them stand out.

Ensuring that their child keeps the hearing aid on was also a source of difficulty for many parents. Some mentioned that children took up to two years to adjust to wearing aids; others developed strategies to ensure the child used the aid.

Children did not often want to wear the aid; at other times they were without them because the aid was broken or was being repaired. Even where the child did wear a hearing aid, this was usually for shorter times than recommended, and often not at home. For some children, aids were only intermittently used, even at school; parents justified this as 'quality time rather than quantity time'.

Overall, parents believed hearing aids to be useful and desirable. However, their views about both the aesthetics and necessity of the hearing aids varied. Some were worried about other children's reactions and bullying in the playground: a concern acutely felt if their child was wearing a bulky aid. Some felt NHS hearing aids were unwieldy and embarrassing; a few bought 'more appropriate', discreet aids.

The most striking disparity between parents' and practitioners' views, however, stemmed from the perceived usefulness and necessity of hearing aids. Two examples illustrate this difference. One mother states that she had been advised by the doctors that the child should wear a hearing aid all the time. She felt, however, that the child could hear without the aid and allowed him to function without it for some of the time. Another mother explained that she was advised to ensure that the aid was used for about two-and-a-half hours each day, which they have done. The mother then said, in contradiction, that the doctors wanted them to ensure that the child wears the hearing aid for the whole day and that it is parents who want their child to wear it for no more than about three hours. The doctors had stated that hearing aids were necessary and they would further help improve the child's speech, which was already relatively well developed. The father also maintained that the local school for deaf children "force you to keep [child's] hearing aids on all the time". Instead, the parents felt that they were better judges of the child's needs than professionals who saw the child briefly and occasionally. They also thought that the child was happier when she was not wearing her aid.

It was suggested earlier that information and advice about hearing aids should take account of parental concerns about amplification support. Parents' views, illustrated above, suggest that there is considerable scope for improving understanding of the utility, efficacy and desirability of hearing aids for the child concerned. Parents do not always accept that wearing hearing aids will enhance sound receptivity and facilitate spoken language. Indeed, some offer reasons suggesting that it hinders the child's development, including speech – these concerns need to be addressed for improved compliance.

## Cochlear implants

On the whole, parents had negative views of cochlear implants. Where parents did consider implants for their child, this was with some ambivalence about their advantages and disadvantages. Parents' knowledge about cochlear implants also varied. Some were well informed, others had only partial or no information. Others still had been told that implants were inappropriate for their child and hence felt no need to know more. For one parent, information about implants was biased: "biased towards going for it and getting it done". This parent's child responded to the most recent hearing test and was told that if the child had a cochlear implant, it would boost the child's hearing; the parent remained ambivalent. However, one parent went on to say: "Having said that, if we think in the long run he's gonna benefit then we'll obviously go for it". Parents offered three main reasons for their reluctance:

- concerns about the surgical procedure and consequent pain;
- worries about a visible scar;
- being unsure if the benefits justified the pain and discomfort to the child.

Some parents were clearly opposed to implants, emphasising their potentially damaging or inconsequential effects, along with the intricacy and length of the operation and the consequent discomfort for the child. These parents appeared to be well informed about implants and had formed their opinions after discussion in the family and with professionals, such as teachers and senior clinical medical officers.

## Language and communication

Here we concentrate on parents' preferences about language and communication for their child.

### Spoken language

A number of parents wanted to support their child in a spoken language as opposed to, or in addition to, sign language. The main justification stemmed from their belief, reinforced or informed by teachers, that this was in the child's best interests. One parent of three children, two of them deaf, wanted her children to learn to speak but would not encourage them in developing spoken language if sign language was going to be the main language at a later point. Other parents wanted children to develop speech as well, but did not feel there was adequate speech and language therapy support, especially in Asian languages.

Professionals had not discussed speech and language therapy with any of these parents, nor had parents, as yet, made enquiries about this themselves. This was partly because speech and language therapy intervention is more common with older children; partly, parents had no reference point with which to gauge service provision and what their child's needs were. Consequently, some parents remained unclear about their child's potential to develop speech. That professionals could not give absolute predictions puzzled these parents.

## Sign language

There was limited support for sign language among this group of parents for a variety of reasons, ranging from parental assessment of the child's hearing to prejudice against sign language and/or views that BSL, and signing in general, was negatively perceived in the Asian community. Most parents would use signing as a last resort but would prefer to concentrate on the child's speech development. In interpreting parental views, it is important to remember they had pre-school children, and issues for older deaf children may be different.

Very few parents expressed positive attitudes towards BSL or wanted their child to rely entirely on sign language. A mother, who supported sign language, explained that although she still wanted her child to learn to lip-read, she thought sign language was very useful. She uses 'own sign language' with the child at home and said that she would learn 'proper' signs when the child was older. She had decided to sign because it made communication with the child easier and valued the pleasure the child was having in being able to communicate. Another parent liked sign language: "because the children get to know, you get what you want, you can understand". However, very few other parents expressed such enthusiasm for sign language.

Parents' views on sign language appear to have been informed, among other things, by professional advice and personal perceptions of what is in their child's best interest. A number of parents, however, expressed concern about their own difficulties in using sign language. Experiences varied. Many did not use or learn sign language at all, while some did. Some expressed a desire for evening sign language classes in their locality. One father expressed reservations about the commitment of other parents, mainly mothers at sign language classes at the local deaf school. He was the only father attending the sign language class and felt that the mothers only went for social reasons, and when transport was provided. This perceived lack of commitment on the part of other parents led him to reduce his attendance from twice to once weekly. The mother of the same child reiterated that her husband felt out of place in this group as no other men attended the group. She helps him with signing and the family have bought various aids to sign language, such as books and videos. Another mother described her enthusiasm for sign language and contrasted this with the reluctance of other family members. Her attempts to persuade her husband to learn signing failed and the wider family did not "speak through signs", leaving her as the main communicator with the child.

## Advice on language and communication

Parents' language preferences for their children were informed by a range of factors such as their religious and cultural persuasions and perceptions of deafness and 'disability'; and also by professional advice. Some felt they were not adequately informed about language choice. One mother stated that she would have welcomed more information about communicating with her child; she was initially bewildered by not knowing what to do. Mothers also felt that the responsibility of communication with children was largely placed on them – fathers and other family members, particularly the extended family, had relatively little interest in learning signing, for example.

If Punjabi or Urdu was the home language, then it was usually advised that the family should communicate with the child in this language, at least in the first instance. Other parents were advised to use signing; information given to parents suggested to them that not to do this would compromise the child's development.

In addition to learning sign language, children were also learning spoken English. Where an Asian language is also spoken at home, particularly when parents do not speak English, the child needs to acquire this language or the parents need to learn English or both need to use sign language. A common scenario was that one or two people in the home became interpreters for the child or parents. It has been argued that some Asian parents of deaf children have been wrongly advised to use only English language with their child even when parents are unable to speak English themselves (see Ahmad et al, in press; Chamba et al, forthcoming: b, for detailed discussion). The main justification for this advice is that it avoids confusion stemming from use of additional language which may compound the child's difficulties with learning spoken language.

Concern about the nature of advice given to parents by health and peripatetic professionals was raised more by practitioners than by parents, and this will be discussed further in Chapter 5. However, one parent raised concerns about appropriateness of advice, its impact on the child's loss of home language and consequent difficulties in communicating with the extended family. Their child was "on the verge of profound deafness and we were advised to not complicate his language development by bringing in bi-lingualism". They used English with the child "and make that his first language". With hindsight, they felt that they were misguided. The family were now helping this child with Urdu but he was "definitely struggling". On discovering that their third child was also deaf, the family decided to use Urdu from the start. Although they initially faced scepticism about their decision, the child now speaks both Urdu and English at a level that "it's enough for him to get on in life".

## Parents' communication strategies

Despite some parents' advocacy of spoken language as opposed to sign language, specific advice given to them about the language in which they should or should not communicate with their child, and parents' personal reservations about, for example, sign language, all parents used a range of languages. No parent relied exclusively on one language.

One parent wanted her child to speak Punjabi when older. Another parent already spoke Punjabi at home with her child, although the child's understanding was better than his speech. The child had also just started picking up English, having started school. Sign language and English played relatively little part in communication where both parents spoke to their child in Punjabi. The child's access to the parental language was perceived to be crucial to family communication and family life more generally.

In other instances, English was preferred and perceived to warrant greater priority. For example, one parent felt that it was more important for a deaf child to learn spoken English because of its closer affinity with lip-reading support (available only in English) and sign language. Similar considerations influenced other parents' choices. For example, as teachers worked with the child in English, the parents also used English. Other parents, in contrast, used a combination of approaches: English, Punjabi and lip-reading; English, Punjabi lip-reading and sign language; "mixed, Punjabi and English, mostly English" lip-reading. Not surprisingly, those parents who doubted the validity of the diagnosis found it more difficult to decide on a communication strategy.

## Peripatetic and other service support

Here we explore parents' experiences of peripatetic and other service support including the information provided to them. The peripatetic service performs a number of important supportive functions for parents and their deaf children. This may include: immediate support after the diagnosis; providing information about voluntary organisations and other agencies; information about the child's deafness; and possible amplification needs, sign language learning and advice on schooling.

Parents expressed general concerns about their child's education. These included worries about the child's educational performance and in one case, lack of staff at the local school for deaf children. More positively, some parents, though expressing concerns about the academic potential of deaf children, were impressed with the 'high educational achievement' of deaf children at one local school for deaf children. Parents complimented this school for the support and advice, the regular visits they received from teachers, the practical help with amplification, support with other aspects of childcare, and the provision of tuition for parents in BSL. They were also comforted by meeting other parents of deaf children at the school. The benefits of such close contact ranged from social support to how to deal better with the deaf child's changing needs, support in their education and development, and practical help with aids and play activities.

As discussed in Chapter 2, early identification of hearing loss needs to be followed by immediate support for parents. Parents complimented the teachers for the range and quality of support following the diagnosis. Parents were also complimentary about specific information that they were given about looking after their deaf child and felt they had received more information from the peripatetic support service than the health service. A comprehensive directory providing information about the range and location of available services was suggested as one helpful approach to information sources.

Translated information and interpreting did not emerge as important issues. This may be partly to do with the fact that about two thirds of the respondents were English speakers. Partly, it may reflect the taken for granted nature of families providing interpreting support themselves. Some respondents, however, felt that interpreting provision would enable them easier access to services. As we will see, professionals were more concerned about inadequate interpreting support (Chapter 6).

## Choice of schooling

The key issue that most parents raised concerned choosing between mainstream and segregated schooling. Parents' views about schooling were informed by factors such as their own language preferences, sign language and other specialist support available in mainstream schools, the degree of the child's deafness, advice from professionals and parents' previous experiences. Parents expressed different views about schooling. A number were in favour of mainstream schools and supporting their child's development in spoken languages, but expressed reservations both about appropriate support in these schools and the prejudice their child might encounter. Many wanted more information about mainstream and specialist schooling before deciding, or wanted the child to attend a school for deaf children when older. Often decisions were finely balanced: perceived advantages and disadvantages of both forms of schooling made decisions difficult. For example, one parent articulated this dilemma in terms of the potential lack of support in a mainstream school but a fear that a "deaf school" may be "just concentrating on his deafness".

The degree of deafness also influenced both advice from teachers and parents' decisions. However, other considerations were also important. For example, one mother preferred her child to attend a mainstream school because he was "picking up words", although the school did not have a deaf unit. The child preferred to go to the current mainstream school because a cousin was also there. The mother's main concern, shared by another parent, was that she did not know if her child was getting any specialist support and wanted a teacher to work with her child. Some parents expressed concern about how their children might be treated if they attended a mainstream school, illustrated by one mother's fears about deaf children being like 'foreigners' in a hearing school and potentially open to bullying.

Although decisions about schooling were mediated through a number of factors, as discussed, we came across very few cases of explicit disagreement between parents and teachers over schooling.

## Voluntary organisations and social services support

Health and education services play the principal role in diagnosis and support, but voluntary organisations and social services also have a potentially important role in services for deaf children.

Parents' understanding and involvement with deaf voluntary organisations varied and generally showed a relative lack of knowledge about their potential role. For example, a mother with a two-year-old deaf child, who had regular visits from peripatetic teachers, did not know about the National Deaf Children's Society and its activities in the area. Other parents had some information about deaf voluntary agencies, Deaf clubs, and parent support groups but would have welcomed a sourcebook which provided all the relevant information in one package. Parents sometimes felt that they were expected to seek relevant information but felt hampered by their lack of awareness of what information or services to ask for and where such information can be obtained.

Even where parents had the relevant information, they did not necessarily use such services. Reasons varied. For example, some preferred to rely on the media, or health and education services for information about deafness rather than on voluntary agencies. Other parents felt that they had considerable family support and therefore did not need to look to voluntary agencies for social support. For others, organised groups were not their 'cup of tea'. Lack of time also made it difficult to attend local social groups.

The level of contact and participation in deaf organisations was limited, but parents' involvement with social services and the level of support from them was even more marginal. The role of social services or a social worker with the deaf was rarely if at all mentioned by parents. Where support from social services was mentioned it was invariably in relation to money and benefits. Support in securing financial aid was much appreciated. Where parents were not receiving allowances they felt they were entitled to, they expressed disappointment or were experiencing hardships. For example, one mother was unhappy about no longer receiving the higher rate of Disability Living Allowance (DLA) and care allowance, after reassessment. Another mother was disappointed with only getting the middle rate of DLA and did not know if she was entitled to any other benefits. She found the Benefits Agency unresponsive to her financial needs, and unsympathetic to claims that it was more expensive to care for her three deaf children than it would be if she had hearing children. She was also dissatisfied with her housing which she felt was unsafe for deaf children. Although she had received considerable support from a social worker with the deaf with her housing worries, it had not made any material difference.

## Other needs and interagency/interprofessional boundaries

As noted, parents have limited contact with voluntary organisations and social services. For social services, this is contrary to what would be expected as community care legislation has given them key responsibility for facilitating interagency collaboration and providing appropriate support for disabled children. This is not being realised in practice and two reasons can be suggested for this. With pre-school deaf children, parents' contact is mainly with health and education services and they may not feel that voluntary organisations and social services have much to offer. It may also be the case that through lack of information and poor interagency collaboration, the potential role of voluntary organisations and social services was not well understood by parents.

Parents' assessment of unmet needs varied. Some parents did not feel that their child needed further support, although need for support in the form of audiological equipment and repairs to aids was mentioned. For example, parents felt that if the audiology department opened for a few hours at weekends, this would enable them to collect items such as batteries. Others felt that help with environmental aids such as flashing door bells and text telephones would help them support older deaf children better. Parents found the demarcation between different agencies and services confusing and unhelpful. Other concerns raised were more intertwined. Some parents felt that the support they required was contingent on their child's development and changing needs as well as their own health and well-being. Further needs related to appropriate housing, household resources, financial aid, safer play facilities for deaf children and items such as televisions with teletext facility. Parents also highlighted the need for financial support with purchasing books and educational toys and videos. Many parents had concerns about housing and environment which were unsafe for deaf children but felt that little support was offered by social services or housing departments. Informal support is discussed in Chapter 4.

## Summary

This chapter has addressed a number of issues around parental contact with services. Parents were generally satisfied with amplification support but many needed more advice and most modified the regime for wearing the aids for a variety of reasons. Parents' decisions on language and communication were often based on limited information, were often finely balanced and related to personal understanding and experience, the nature of the child's deafness and professional advice. Contact with the peripatetic teachers was highly valued, particularly the coordinating role performed by teachers. Social services and the voluntary sector played more peripheral roles. There was generally good interagency collaboration between health and education but interagency working between health and social services and the voluntary sector was less well developed.

# FOUR

# The family and social context

Previous chapters have focused on parents' experiences of formal support from health, education, social services and voluntary organisations. The caring role is largely performed by parents and other members of the immediate family while the wider family context is important in the child's development and furnishing a supportive environment. This chapter focuses on the parental and wider family's role in relation to young deaf children: how they share information, their own knowledge and perceptions of deafness, the reactions of family members to diagnosis and forms of family support. We consider the caring role, largely performed by parents, but in which the wider family can act as a significant resource. Knowledge and perceptions about deafness are explored before considering how these relate to aspects of ethnicity, culture and religion. Finally, we turn to what parents' advice would be to other parents with young deaf children and explore their perspectives and concerns in relation to their deaf child's future life.

## Telling the family

Deafness may already be anticipated by the wider family and friends as they may have shared, or indeed contributed to, the parents' suspicions and concerns before a formal diagnosis. Parents' feelings about telling other people, particularly outside the immediate family, are shaped by their views about their child's deafness, attitudes to disability and anticipation of others' reactions. Most shared the diagnosis with members of their family as well as non-kin, although the place and timing of such disclosures was important and varied between parents. For example, parents preferred to discuss the diagnosis in a face-to-face meeting, especially with close kin. It was also easier to tell other people after the parents themselves had come to terms with the diagnosis. Some parents found it more difficult to tell the family than friends, but it was felt that the former had a right to know and they were kept updated, usually after each of the child's appointments. However, in some cases there was an initial reluctance to sharing such information with others, including wider family.

# Family reaction to the diagnosis

Parents' views about disclosure of diagnosis to others may have been influenced by the anticipated reaction of other people. In some instances, the reaction of family and close friends was supportive, and parents were less concerned about the reaction of distant relatives. Work colleagues were also seen to be supportive. Some attempted to conceal the child's deafness from grandparents and other family abroad who, they thought, would find the news distressing. On the other hand, in families with a history of deafness, there was an easier acceptance of deafness by older family members, representing a negotiated understanding at family level.

A common familial reaction was one of disbelief or denial, not dissimilar to parents' own reactions to the diagnosis. In some cases, the wider family found it difficult to accept the diagnosis because it did not accord with their own assessment. In other cases, different family members had different responses. For other children, the parents' reservations about the accuracy of the diagnosis were also shared by other family members.

## Effect on the family

In most cases families did not function as homogenous entities; different family members played different roles in relation to the child. In some cases, the family members adjusted to the diagnosis relatively quickly. Families with a history of deafness found adjustment easier. For example, one mother described how her in-laws have found it easier to manage their grandchild's deafness than herself because of a history of deafness in her husband's family. In other cases, relatives found the episode traumatic and difficult to adjust to; and in some cases the parents supported other family members in coming to terms with the diagnosis. Many parents reported considerable family support: in some cases, family members were concerned to learn sign language to facilitate family communication with the deaf child.

However, the wider family is not always found to be helpful. Some found the family's reaction unhelpful, which added to their existing worries. They resented this as they felt that the child's deafness had implications largely for their own lives and not for the lives of the wider family. Equally, some were troubled by the unhelpful (compensatory) attention their deaf children received from relatives, which they saw as leaving them with 'spoilt children' to cope with.

Apportioning blame to a spouse or other family members for the child's deafness did not feature in the parents' accounts. In addition to feeling that responsibility for providing support resided mainly with the parents, on the whole, parents also felt that having a deaf child did not, as some may expect, bring the family closer together. Apart from the use of sign language – even here, not all families or members within a family participated equally (but in a few cases members of the extended family had acquired some signing skills) – relationships and responsibilities had remained largely as before. In some cases parents felt more responsible and 'grown up' as a consequence of having a deaf child. Noting these experiences is important as they contest the commonly-held view that Asian families necessarily 'look after their own' or do not welcome support beyond the family.

## Family support and advice for parents

A wide range of lay, familial, medical and educational advice and knowledge inform parental views about deafness and future course of action. Their views and experiences are mediated by, among other factors, a history of deafness within the family, the composition of individuals in the household, parental and other family obligations and the geographical proximity of the immediate or extended family members.

A number of parents with deaf children also had relatives with deaf children. For example, in one case a close relative had four deaf children and in another, three out of eight children were deaf. Such families had greater knowledge, experience and skills to draw on than families with no recent history of deafness. Household composition varied enormously, from the nuclear to extended families. A number of parents had next of kin within a comfortable distance. In nuclear families, parents of deaf children often had relatives nearby who saw children daily; some visited frequently but not daily; others lived next door and were able to give practical support whenever needed. However, the mundane and routine care rested predominantly with parents, generally the mother, with varying degrees of support from their husbands, sisters, child's grandparents and other relatives.

## Caring for a deaf child

Parents remain the principal care-givers of deaf children. Support from health, education, other services and from other family members can considerably help with caring responsibilities. Here we address the difficulties that parents continue to experience in caring, followed by looking at those aspects in which they feel they and their children require further support.

### 'Good' and 'bad' experiences of looking after a deaf child

Parents had both 'good' and 'bad' experiences of caring for their deaf children; not surprisingly, many of the problems were those generally experienced by parents of young children. Equally, parents commented positively on the child's endearing qualities and took pleasure in the child's achievements, such as in learning sign language. Some felt that having a deaf child provided them with important insights into the lives and needs of disabled people and their families.

A majority of parents felt that caring for their deaf child presented additional difficulties. The main difficulty that parents expressed related to communication which either made certain tasks harder, required being more attentive to the child's needs, or made mutual understanding between the family and child difficult. For example, because of relatively poor communication between parents and children some parents were confused about whether the child did not understand or whether they were 'playing up'. Sometimes a child would throw tantrums, initiated or exacerbated by problems in communication. Parents also confronted additional physical demands imposed by caring for their deaf child as it was necessary to be much more attentive to the child's needs and their 'misdemeanours'. For example, a mother talked of the need to be with the child much more and its impact on reducing her social life as well as opportunities for paid work, neither of which were affected to the same degree by her previous (hearing) children.

Caring tasks which parents mentioned as problematic included persistence with hearing aids, because the child found it difficult to get used to them, and helping the child to dress, an activity which the parents felt would be performed relatively easily with a hearing child. Some parents found the additional responsibility related to having a deaf child, such as going to the local school for deaf children, learning sign language and attending appointments, difficult to cope with. Parents also projected concerns about changing issues which will confront themselves or their children as the children grow older, such as the child wishing to be 'normal' and the problems this created. For example, one parent talked of her older deaf child denying his deafness and refusing to use his hearing aid in an attempt to be "accepted as a normal person".

# Knowledge and perceptions of deafness

Parents' knowledge and perceptions of deafness informed their contact with services before, during and after the diagnosis. A discussion of parents' knowledge and perceptions of deafness and the Deaf community, and how they thought Asian cultures perceive deafness provides an important context for understanding both their perspectives, and interaction with services. Parents' views suggest that ethnicity, religion, and previous history of deafness in the family are important factors in their views on deafness and disability.

Parents varied in deaf awareness. Some were well informed, including having good knowledge of the Deaf community and culture, and BSL skills and wanted their children to be involved with the Deaf community. In most cases, however, their previous knowledge of deafness was confined to knowing individual hard of hearing adults or deaf children in the family or among acquaintances. Much of the parents' knowledge about deafness and Deaf culture was acquired through the peripatetic teachers, and in some cases through personal reading. Few had contact with Asian deaf adults.

Not surprisingly, parents' views changed over time. One mother initially felt that deaf people had limited communication skills and a bleak future, but following a visit to the local school for deaf children she was more positive. On learning about her own child's deafness, she remembered negative perceptions of deafness in Pakistan, but her doctor reassured her that attitudes in Britain were more positive and facilities were better. The mother's main concern at the time of the interview was to ensure that her child went to the right school. In a different vein, a father, himself disabled, did not think that his wife's experience of having a deaf child had changed her attitude – her expectations remained low.

Some parents saw deaf children or adults as 'normal' apart from their hearing, and located their deafness in nature or divine will. The tendency to emphasise 'normalcy' is a common response of parents of disabled or chronically ill children, who 'normalise' the children by discounting the disability and concentrating on other aspects of the child's lives. Others expressed major concerns about the child's deafness and its implications for the future, fearing that the child would need support throughout their life, which may not be available after the parents' death.

## Ethnicity and culture

The perceived importance of ethnicity featured quite often in parents' accounts when they were asked how they felt Asian people viewed deafness. Views on deafness differed. Some felt that Asian people held less negative views about deafness than the white population. The perception that deafness (or disability) has less negative connotations, however, was not widely shared. A number of parents felt that Asian people perceived deafness negatively; feeling sorry for deaf children and giving them 'extra love' reflected this. In the experience of some parents, Asian people looked down on deaf people and would stare at a deaf child with a hearing aid, while white people would not. They argued that this difference stemmed from Asian people's reluctance to accept disability and manifested itself in the patronising treatment of parents and deaf children.

These perceived negative views manifested in apathy, and viewing the deaf child as a burden. The resources available to support deaf children and their families were thus not always utilised by parents. A mother, active in deaf voluntary organisations, emphasised the range of facilities and benefits available for deaf children in Britain and compared these to the lack of support in Pakistan, stressing the need for parents to become better informed, motivated and to use available support for their own and their child's benefit. Another parent felt, however, that although people continue to be patronising and ignorant, perceptions of deafness were becoming less negative.

## The importance of religion

Not only is religion complexly interwoven with culture, gender and ethnicity, its relationship to views about deafness and disability also varies for different parents. This suggests that even for a group of people who were relatively homogenous in terms of religion and ethnicity, the precise role, significance and implications of religion can be different.

A number of parents were explicit about what they wanted in terms of religious education. They wanted their child to learn about religion either at home or by attending the mosque, especially to learn to read the Quran. Many stressed instilling culturally and religiously appropriate gender values as a particularly important aspect of religious education. Ideally, for some parents, schools should also take an interest in stressing religious and cultural values. Parents had varying degrees of confidence in the ability and willingness of schools to do this.

Religion also provided the basis of coping with deafness and accepting responsibilities as parents. As Allah was perceived to be accountable for determining people's destinies, their child's deafness was predetermined. However, this 'fatalism' was coupled with a sense of God-given responsibility to do the best for their child. A belief in the role of God in life and its struggles helped parents to come to terms with their child's deafness.

In contrast to these parents, some with more secular views expressed concern about those with religious convictions. While respecting the meaning that religion gives to people, their views suggested that religion encouraged complacent attitudes towards deafness rather than proactive and supportive responses. On the whole, however, parents used religion as a flexible resource which was inextricably linked to social, cultural and gender identity, and which enabled acceptance of deafness and emphasised the need to do the best for their child.

## The future

Reflecting on their overall experiences of caring for a deaf child and contact with services, parents expressed a wide range of hopes and fears about the immediate and distant future. Parents, particularly those with children with additional disabilities, hoped that their child's physical development would improve, that they would acquire an understanding of their religion and culture, attain greater 'normality', improve communication skills in sign and speech and hope that their child would be able to do what they want. One of the parents' principal concerns was for children to start a deaf nursery at an early age and progress to a school with support for deaf children and ultimately perform well academically and in employment.

Parents expressed concern about what the child would be like when older. Other concerns related to the child's ability to cope with independent life, improvement in coping with deafness, child safety, and the need to challenge disablism, particularly in employment. One mother raised concerns about her family doctor's ability to communicate with her child and know her child's background. There was concern about perceived falling educational standards and in one locality, the shortage of staff in a local school for deaf children. Very few parents stated that they had no concerns for the future.

## Advice for other parents

Parents suggested a wide range of issues when considering the advice they would volunteer to other parents of a newly-diagnosed deaf child. Advice offered was contingent on the age and individual needs of the child. Respondents felt that if a parent is suspicious about hearing loss, they should contact services straight away and have the child's hearing checked quickly. Once the child is diagnosed, parents should obtain as much information as possible, as not all relevant information may have been given by professionals. It was also important to ask questions and pursue all avenues of potential support. It was imperative that all tests were done effectively to facilitate earlier diagnosis.

They felt that parents should ensure that doctors listen to what they have to say, as parents often know what is best, and learn to accept their child's deafness quickly to ensure appropriate support for the child. It was felt to be important not to treat your newly-diagnosed deaf child differently to a hearing child, to give the child time to develop and to get used to the child's deafness and not to underestimate their potential in education and employment. Taking an active role was felt to be important "because at end of day you've [parents] got to communicate with your child". For this reason, most felt that it was important to learn sign language, especially those who had followed this option themselves, although mothers were more proactive than fathers.

## Summary

The reactions of the wider family to diagnosis were often similar to those of parents. Some parents found the wider family supportive, while a few complained of little positive support but unhelpful indulgence of the deaf child, which created problems for parents. Caring was largely the mothers' responsibility who, compared to fathers and other family members, were also more concerned to ensure good communication with the deaf child. Parents were concerned about the limited knowledge as well as negative attitudes in relation to deafness both within the Asian and the white populations. Religion was used by many parents as a flexible coping resource which facilitated adjustment while at the same time heightening a sense of responsibility to achieve the best for the deaf child.

# FIVE

# Professionals' perspectives: screening and diagnosis

Parents' initial contact with hospital or community based services is concerned with audiological assessment and establishing the existence and degree of hearing loss and appropriate amplification support. Parents may come into contact with a wide range of professionals including health visitors, GPs, senior clinical medical officers, consultant ENT surgeons, paediatric audiological technicians and community paediatricians. The peripatetic support service may also be involved during and following the diagnosis. In exploring practitioners' views and experiences of working with Asian families with a deaf child, a number of distinct issues and concerns have emerged, many of which are often shared by parents of children with other disabilities (Beresford et al, 1996).

This chapter focuses on the coordination of services, screening, epidemiology and early identification of childhood hearing impairment, and causation. Chapter 6 considers views on how services can be improved. To some extent the organisation of material into these two chapters is for convenience and the reader is advised to read both chapters for an understanding of professionals' accounts.

## Service coordination and interagency collaboration

Professionals from different agencies work with deaf children and their families. Service coordination was a long-standing concern for purchasers and providers in this study. Problems can arise both between agencies and between different professionals within the same agency. Practitioners' views about the quality, efficiency and coordination of services were contingent upon their location, the local service context, and recent changes in service organisation. For example, this research coincided with changes taking place within one locality which involved the integration of an audiology department with the ENT service in the same hospital and closer collaboration with the peripatetic education service. The consultant

ENT surgeon felt the integration would allow an improved service.

In most study sites there were better working relationships between health and education services than between health and social services. However, social services often worked closely with the education sector. Social services professionals were concerned about health visitors, GPs, teachers and other professionals performing the social worker's role, without the requisite training or knowledge, an issue also raised by some teachers and health visitors. The need for closer collaboration between education and social services was emphasised by social service respondents as teachers were not perceived to have the professional remit or skills to provide emotional support or help with benefits, adaptations and equipment. An agreed protocol for interagency work and for cross-referrals was regarded to be important. This would ensure that the wider needs of the family, including social and emotional support, and access to benefits and equipment, were addressed through referrals to social services and other agencies. One locality had established a liaison group composed of members from social services, education, health services and the voluntary sector to encourage closer working. However, the need to change attitudes to interagency collaboration was emphasised: a social services respondent, for example, felt colleagues in the education service were 'secretive' about sharing information, to the detriment of a coordinated and comprehensive service. Purchasers felt that social services only had a limited role to play with young deaf children although their role became more important as children became older or when they had other needs.

Problems of coordination are not confined to interagency working. A health visitor gave the example of a family who could name about six different health visitors they had contact with in the previous six months. Health visitors also noted poor communication between themselves and other health professionals. For example, they felt that keeping abreast with individual children's progress through health services would be easier if they, like GPs, were routinely informed, about "what goes [on] in hospitals".

It was anticipated, however, that the integration of services across specialties and agencies would have many benefits, a view purchasers shared. It would:

- allow a central database and facilitate targeting 'at-risk' families;
- reduce the costs of running an audiological service;
- improve the statementing process;
- facilitate information sharing;
- be less confusing for parents.

The relationship with the peripatetic support service, often based in the local schools for deaf children, and community paediatricians and physicians was thought to be already excellent.

The need for a coordinated approach was illustrated by a teacher who highlighted the problems of some families with more than one child having to attend two separate hospitals about 10 miles apart, based in separate provider trusts, for different children. One possible reason for this was that some consultants worked between the two trusts and divided their workload, which was confusing for parents and difficult to understand for other professionals. The main difficulties faced by parents related to transport and coordination of childcare, especially where there were young children of different ages. This, according to some professionals, led to difficulties in keeping appointments, and an overall inadequate service for parents.

In an attempt to ensure better collaboration between professionals, home visits were often made by health and education professionals together. On the surface, this had many benefits in providing a coordinated service. However, when they were also accompanied by interpreters, it was felt that the presence of three or more professionals in the house at the same time was perhaps overpowering for many families.

There was also concern about coordination in a sizeable town with a well-established Asian population. One senior clinical medical officer described the importance of involving a wide range of professionals, including multilingual speech therapists and educational social workers. Problems included:

- poor information sharing;
- lack of an agreed protocol;
- poor understanding of the audiological service by managers.

According to this senior clinical medical officer, these professionals' "ears are not audiologically tuned". The senior clinical medical officer felt that clear responsibility for coordinated services resting with one named individual would facilitate an improved service which was responsive and based on identified need, something also highlighted by other professionals. The service needed to be based on local and national evidence rather than on historical precedence or personal preferences of practitioners.

Some of these views were also echoed by practitioners in a large city with well-established services for deaf people. While there was perceived to be a good level of integration and cooperation in this area, there was both room for improvement and a realisation that services for deaf people may be seen as low priority within a fierce competition for resources in the health services. A poorly integrated service also meant duplication (eg, hospital and community audiology). Within this locality, services are available at about a dozen different clinics. Although offering easier access, it resulted in other difficulties such as problems of central records, lack of secretarial support, and difficulty in providing a comprehensive service at so many different sites.

Some practitioners felt that inequalities in access had been exacerbated by the changes in primary healthcare following the 1990s reforms, to the detriment of minority ethnic patients. Examples of 'unfairness' included fundholding GPs being able to make direct referrals to consultants, thus adversely affecting the length of time other parents have to wait for a hospital appointment. Recognising this as unfair, some professionals helped parents 'play this game' to 'short circuit' the system.

## Genetic counselling

Access to genetic counselling service was perceived to suffer particularly from poor coordination. Many professionals felt that not enough referrals were being made by audiological services, especially by ENT surgeons. Reasons included:

- services being divided between acute and community trusts with no clear protocols for referrals;
- lack of guidance from purchasers and managers on referral policy.

The implications of such inadequacies are that parents may be denied access to information which they may value, and genetic counselling was a well-established regional resource with both practice and research expertise.

Because of the relatively poor referrals system, most families were being referred when the child was two or three years old and in some cases the family would already have younger deaf children. According to one senior practitioner and researcher in genetics, only about 5% of the families with two or more deaf children were being referred to genetic counselling service. This practitioner emphasised that purchasers and providers needed to recognise the potential benefits of ongoing developments in molecular genetics, although this would impose further strains on resources.

Others, while recognising under-referral, felt that there had been some improvements. Different explanations for underutilisation were offered. Some felt it was a failure on the part of community paediatricians. One consultant who was convinced of the link between consanguineous marriages and deafness and attributed failure to attend appointments entirely to parents, also felt it would be difficult to encourage Asian parents to attend for genetic counselling. In one of the areas, social services staff as well as others were making some referrals to genetic counselling.

Need for greater involvement by public health and health promotion to raise awareness of diseases which caused deafness and of the importance of early referral for genetic counselling was also emphasised. In addition, another practitioner pointed to the need to dispense stereotyped assumptions (sometimes also held by Asian practitioners) about, for example, Muslim parents being 'fatalistic', which may lead to parents not being offered a service.

Among purchasers, there was no consensus on the utility of genetic counselling. One purchaser, for example, felt that perhaps too many referrals were being made in their locality. Another, from a city with a large Asian population and which has considerably greater proportional referral rates for genetic counselling, believed that the growth of the Asian population as a proportion of the total population and advances in genetics will make genetic counselling even more relevant in years to come. However, other purchasers felt that until the predictive ability of genetic counselling improved, it would remain of limited value.

## Screening children for hearing loss

While the importance of child health surveillance and screening is not in dispute, the nature, frequency and cost-effectiveness of screening procedures is contested among paediatric professionals, including health visitors. One thrust behind the Hall Report was that practitioners should use less screening and do it better (Hall, 1991). This was felt to be problematic by some health visitors, because a number of children with 'borderline' hearing loss were picked up at around the age of three years. The health visitors felt that abandoning the functional tests would mean many deaf children not being identified and offered support. The gap between tests at seven to eight months and when children start nursery was perceived as too long by some health visitors.

However, there was no consensus among professionals; a range of views were held about screening. *Universal* neonatal screening was one important issue to emerge, although views on this differed. Some emphasised that even if universal screening could be instituted, there would still be a need for additional screening to identify:

- children 'who deteriorated' but were fine at the earlier tests;
- children with significant conductive hearing loss;
- children who moved into the area.

However, there were further problems with the neonatal screening tests which related to false positives and false negatives. For example many children do not 'pass' because they have fluid in the ear and as they have to come back, this puts strain on the system. Further, while universal neonatal screening may be desirable it may not be possible practically or financially.

*At-risk screening* was proposed as a more cost-effective compromise and commended where it was already in place. However, a standard protocol for at-risk registers was deemed important. The at-risk register in one of the cities allowed detection of two or more deaf children per 1,000, children were diagnosed within three months and as such the screening was perceived to be successful. It was recognised that such screening can never be 100% effective as children often acquired hearing problems after the screening, as well as for other reasons. It was still important to rely on information given by parents as they were seen to be important instigators of the diagnostic process.

Reservations were expressed about the introduction of further screening in addition to at-risk registers. Various reasons were offered for this. One practitioner was unsure if it mattered whether a child was identified at eight weeks or eight months; thus, having additional tests designed to identify deafness earlier would be of dubious value. Others felt that further screening tests would add little. Assuming that at-risk screening identified 50% of the deaf children and a further 30-40% were identified by distraction tests, it was felt that not many tests are good enough to match the coverage provided by existing methods (ie, around 80-90%). In addition, children were also being identified through school medical examinations at the age of six. Some felt that considerable benefits could be achieved through improved use of existing systems, and an improved at-risk register and referral system, without instituting additional tests or universal screening.

## The distraction test

The distraction test is a central element of screening. Important issues include the relationship between parents and health visitors, difficulties in assessing language development and other problems related to the distraction test itself.

For some professionals, health service changes created additional worries. A community paediatrician felt, for example, that a major worry nationally was that, due to GP fundholding, health visitors would not be allowed to refer by traditional routes. Beyond diagnosis, it was felt that health visitors should attend to general medical problems and parents' queries about deafness should be dealt with by teachers. Health visitors acknowledged parents' complaints about their limited involvement beyond diagnosis. The health visiting role was perceived as flexible, difficult to define precisely and difficult for parents to understand. The generic role of health visitors was valued by parents, as described in Chapter 2. Other professionals complimented health visitors for facilitating the referral process and helping to reduce the rates of non-attendance by contacting audiology departments directly and recommending that a test should be done immediately, when, for example, it became known that parents would be going to Pakistan. In some cases, health visitors were also sent a copy of the appointment letter and contacted again if the parent and child failed to attend.

As noted, health visitors raised concerns about the circumstances under which distraction tests were conducted. Lack of soundproof rooms meant that tests were being conducted against varying degrees of background noise, exacerbated also by the child being accompanied by other siblings; this applied both to tests conducted in homes as well as in clinics.

In addition to the environment, health visitors as well as other professionals emphasised the importance of the health visitors having the necessary training and skills in conducting the test. Some health visitors felt that financial constraints were preventing refresher training and updating of skills.

A further problem noted by health visitors and others was the non-Asian professionals' difficulty in assessing the language development of young children who do not use English, and some children's "unfamiliarity with white faces". This was perceived to hinder adequate testing of children aged around 18 months, when children start using spoken language. Further, professionals' possible low expectations about speech development of Asian children may influence the efficiency with which language development is assessed.

Concerns about the usefulness of this test and the skills of the health visitor were raised by other practitioners, including concerns about training and where and how referrals were made. The latter was particularly important for one locality where there was no explicit district-wide policy on paediatric audiology. However, many felt that despite the difficulties with distraction tests, health visitors played a vital role in detecting deafness.

## Epidemiology and late diagnosis

The quality and appropriateness of services is, to a large extent, contingent upon practitioners' knowledge of the demographic and epidemiological profile of the local population and the extent to which this knowledge is translated into the organisation of services. It is therefore important to discuss practitioners' knowledge of the population and how this influenced services. Professionals differed in their views about epidemiology of childhood deafness. Views about whether Asian deaf children were diagnosed later than white children also differed. Some emphasised the unique demographic and epidemiological profile of certain localities within West Yorkshire and the implications of this for health and education services.

Professionals generally felt that there was a proportionately higher number of Asian children who were deaf; they noted this in relation to the number of Asian deaf children in nurseries, although some remained unconvinced in the absence of sound epidemiological data. On the whole, practitioners did not draw links between demography, epidemiology and late diagnosis. The demography and epidemiology of childhood hearing impairment were seen as a separate issue from whether Asian children were being diagnosed later due to inaccessible services. While practitioners raised discrete issues around, for example, appointments, the distraction test, need for interpreters and problems of access, there was no explicit reference to the possible cumulative effect of these factors on diagnosis.

Practitioners differed in their views about possible 'late diagnosis' of Asian deaf children. Some felt that this was no longer the case – in particular, the at-risk register in one of the localities, it was felt, ensured speedy testing of babies born in families with a history of deafness. To some, improvements in the time taken to reach diagnosis had taken place in all the study sites. For babies in 'at-risk' families, diagnoses were usually made within six to eight weeks. Indeed, some felt that Asian children were diagnosed at a younger age compared to white children. However, some health visitors feared that over-reliance on at-risk registers may deflect attention away from children born in families where there is no history of deafness. Technical as well as resource issues also made more comprehensive screening a less attractive option. There was not perceived to be an ethnic difference in being on the at-risk register, where such registers were functioning. However, a high rate of non-attendance at appointments and missing distraction tests among Asian parents, sometimes due to extended visits abroad, were seen as potential reasons for delays in the diagnostic process (but see discussion in Chapter 6).

For some, communication problems played an important part in presumed late diagnosis. Others implicated cultural differences in attitudes to deafness as well as stereotypes held by some professionals of what an appropriate level of language development for similarly aged children from different cultural groups may be. While most respondents were satisfied with the speed with which diagnoses were made once parents accessed services, there were reservations about the role of primary healthcare practitioners in terms of limited specialist knowledge of deafness, fears that practitioners did not take parental concerns seriously, and lack of language support for parents, especially the Bangladeshi population.

Finally, children with complex or multiple disabilities were perceived to be less easy to diagnose quickly.

## Causation and consanguinity

A major concern for parents, after the diagnosis, was for meaningful information about why their child was deaf and the implications of the child's hearing impairment for future language development. Practitioners stated that it was often difficult to know the cause at the time of the diagnosis or to predict the precise outcome. However, some still felt that the consultants should discuss the likely cause with parents, and ensure that, if appropriate, they are referred to genetic counselling. In many practitioners' views, there was a strong genetic basis to hearing loss among Asian children.

Consanguinity featured as a major explanation for deafness in Asian children among health visitors as well as other professionals. However, some believed this more strongly than others. The need to address the issue further was reiterated by some practitioners who suggested that it is not possible to conclude, on the basis of the available evidence, that consanguinity is the only, or predominant factor involved in the higher incidence of deafness. The importance of other factors such as vaccination, environmental causes, socioeconomic factors and differential morbidity patterns among Asian women which may contribute to the higher incidence of hearing impairment also needed to be acknowledged. Parents' views about causation, and the potential role of consanguinity, are discussed in Chapter 4.

## Summary

This chapter has explored service coordination within and between agencies, genetic counselling provision, screening, distraction tests, concerns about late diagnosis and professionals' views about causation of deafness among Asian children. Service coordination differed between areas and agencies. In most localities there were strong links between health and education services; links with social services and the voluntary sector were poor. The relatively poor use of the well-resourced regional genetic counselling service was bemoaned by some. Reasons given for lack of referrals included the division of audiology services between acute and community sectors, lack of clear guidance on referrals and questions on the utility of genetic counselling in reducing childhood deafness. Few believed that universal screening would improve coverage; an intelligent use of the at-risk register combined with distraction tests was felt to provide sufficient coverage.

# SIX

# Professionals' perspectives: improving services

A number of areas central to improving healthcare for young deaf children are explored in this chapter. Having an efficient and user-friendly appointments system is central to ensuring access to services. We have explored parents' concerns; here we discuss practitioners' views on appointments and the means of improving attendance. Access to health and other services remains a major problem for significant numbers of minority ethnic people (Hopkins and Bahl, 1993) and for minority ethnic deaf people (Ahmad et al, 1998). We discuss access to health and education services: information, disclosure, accessibility, and communication and interpretation. We then explore practitioners' views about amplification support. Finally, we examine commissioners' accounts about purchasing and contracting and their views about an 'ideal service'.

## Improving attendance at appointments

There was broad agreement that failure to keep appointments posed problems. A number of reasons were given for non-attendance, mainly due to organisational failures:

- language difficulties and lack of interpreters;
- appointments in different localities without good reasons;
- frequent and often late changes to appointments;
- childcare problems.

Others argued that missed appointments were confined predominantly to Asian parents; further, one practitioner believed that there was a gender bias with appointments more likely to be kept for boys than for girls. However, often practitioners, particularly health visitors and teachers, although agreeing that missed appointments were a problem, felt that they were not confined to Asian parents. Health visitors added to the reasons for non-attendance given above, which applied equally to white parents:

- the concerned person not picking up the appointment letter;
- letters going astray as people move house;
- the distance to travel to hospital.

Indeed, Asian parents were felt, by some, to try harder to keep in touch, but were disadvantaged by a potentially inhospitable service. Although sometimes prolonged visits to Pakistan caused disruption, some professionals remarked that this did not explain the problem of missed appointments. Equally, parents' commitment to the service was exemplified by the fact that often they were in touch with the service immediately on their return from Pakistan.

A particular potential cause of parental resentment, and of missed appointments, was given as *block bookings*. Purchasers felt resolution of the problems with appointments rested with the provider and the system needed to improve to meet the Patients' Charter criteria. However, some practitioners suggested that there were parents who were less committed to using available services for their children without additional help, such as with transport. It was suggested that more locally-based clinics, to cut down on travel, and extra administrative staff to facilitate greater compliance with appointments may help.

Language was perceived to be one of the factors which hindered parents attending appointments. Professionals in some areas requested that parents attending their first appointments should bring someone with them to interpret. Interpreters were somewhat easier to arrange for subsequent appointments, although it still led to considerable delays. Translating letters into relevant languages was also suggested, but faced the difficulty of not always knowing which was the appropriate language for the parents concerned. We return to this later.

Poor collaboration and coordination created additional problems. Parents often had as many as four appointments to attend in different places (sometimes different trusts) over a matter of a few days, made more difficult by appointments not taking into account schooling arrangements. Moreover, they were often compelled to take other children out of school because of childcare difficulties or often to help with interpreting. Further, the frequency with which appointments were changed was seen by some practitioners as a major contributory factor to missed appointments. According to one practitioner, this happens so frequently that parents "no longer write it on the calendar", believing it is likely to change again. Poor administrative practice was felt to be behind these changes to appointments. As one practitioner explained, appointment clerks are not always sure about the consultants' availability and book appointments on the basis of partial information. Some practitioners also expressed concerns about parents not being offered a follow-up appointment if they missed two appointments, unless they sought another referral to audiology. At worst, parents were 'struck off'.

A small number of practitioners argued that cultural practices about gender roles and seclusion were responsible for missed appointments. On the other hand, other practitioners appealed for greater cultural sensitivity and more bilingual support. This was exemplified in the comments of a teacher who emphasised the dangers of cultural stereotyping and the need to reach out to the community rather than engage in victim blaming.

## Access to health, education and social services

Practitioners raised a number of issues related to working with Asian families, such as access to information, clearer and empathetic disclosure, a need for greater assertiveness on the part of parents and better interpreting and communication.

### Information and disclosure of diagnosis

Parents were often felt to be poorly informed – a factor related to language problems, non-availability of translated materials and lack of bilingual staff. Efforts were being made in some of the areas to develop and translate materials in the main Asian languages, especially Urdu.

Practitioners felt that parents wanted to know more about what to expect in consultations as this helped to alleviate anxiety and enabled them to prepare for hospital meetings and to think of relevant questions to ask. There were different opinions about who should take responsibility for explaining tests but a consensus that the peripatetic support service should maintain a strong role in this alongside the consultant. In other areas, consultants played a stronger role in disclosure and follow-up information, although not always successfully, according to one senior health practitioner: "It's the role of the consultants here, but I think they fail miserably like all consultants do".

The teachers' involvement in diagnosis and information-giving was not uniform across areas. In one locality, teachers had a more limited role in the diagnostic process and the need for closer involvement was emphasised. The role of social services overlaps with many of the functions performed by other practitioners, an issue noted in Chapter

5. Social services professionals emphasised the need to inform 'the public' of their role. They feared that parents "see social workers like having horns". To make themselves accessible, an attempt was being made in some areas to function through Centres for the Deaf or in collaboration with voluntary agencies.

The disclosure represents the culmination of often a series of hearing tests and needs to be handled sensitively. We noted earlier that some parents were dissatisfied with the disclosure, dissatisfaction arising from the brevity of consultations, the perceived unsympathetic attitude of the consultants and lack of opportunity to ask questions. It was therefore important to have teachers present at the diagnostic consultation so that they could provide a counselling role. Not all areas had close working arrangements between health and education services. Further, the lack of appropriate facilities was felt to hamper the provision of a more sensitive service. This included basic problems of not having a room in which to have a private meeting. At times, teachers counselled and comforted often distraught parents in busy hospital corridors.

Practitioners acknowledged parents' concerns for clearer information about deafness. It was also noted that parents needed to be informed about how high frequency loss could remain undetected until quite late, and given an idea about what to look for in identifying such hearing loss. It was also held that Asian parents tended not to ask questions, which practitioners related to the parents' inability to speak English. Practitioners felt that parents needed to be more assertive in their dealings with professionals if they wished to obtain the information they wanted, a suggestion also made by some parents.

## Accessibility

Other suggestions about improving access included locally-based services which avoid problems of transport. However, elsewhere we have noted the concerns of some practitioners about such a service being overstretched, fragmented and creating problems of coordination. Many professionals emphasised the need for more bilingual staff; this would ease problems of access, particularly poor communication and provide access to vital information for parents.

Other health visitors emphasised the importance of supporting parents in a variety of areas to ensure a good service: by providing support to cope with the diagnosis, information about deafness, practical help with benefits and allowances, help with education resources, and answering parents' questions on child development. Social services can play a potentially important role here. The need to set the deaf child's needs in the wider context of development, family support, benefits and equipment was raised by social services staff, as noted in Chapter 5. In one locality, social services were working with the National Deaf Children's Society to develop an 'advocacy scheme' to act as a 'one-stop shop', allowing people access to a variety of resources and information. However, the generally poor relationship between health and social services in services for deaf children meant that few health professionals mentioned any such involvement from social services.

## Communication and interpreting

As we noted in earlier chapters, very few parents raised the lack of interpreting support as an issue. This contrasts with practitioners' views, suggesting that more support is required.

Poor communication due to language differences was perceived by practitioners, especially health visitors and teachers, but also by social services professionals, to be a major problem in ensuring a mutually productive exchange between themselves and parents. Teachers, often left to 'pick up the pieces', commented in greater detail on the necessity of good interpreting support and having more bilingual professionals; sentiments mirrored also in health visitors' comments. The Single Regeneration Budget (SRB) had renewed funding for a bilingual worker in one locality for a further three years but there was greater concern elsewhere. Concerns were strong in one locality with a large Asian population, where the historical and demographic profile would suggest that an interpreting service should be an integral and well-established feature of the health service. Although the trust had a liaison officer scheme, it was overstretched and the audiology service did not have a dedicated interpreting service. Generic interpreters did not have a detailed knowledge of deaf services. While the identification of deaf children through the at-risk register was perceived to be successful, it was felt that parents were not always fully informed due to poor communication. Access to interpreters was poor in hospitals and somewhat better in the community. Quality of interpreting, and training of both interpreters and those who work with them were raised as issues. Mothers, who were more likely to need interpreters than fathers, were seen to be particularly disadvantaged because of the inadequate interpreting provision.

Purchasers' views on interpreting services differed. One argued for a well-resourced central interagency provision, available to services ranging from probation to audiology and including the voluntary sector. This contradicts the views of some practitioners who emphasised the importance of accessibility, detailed knowledge of the service, rapport with other professionals, and good awareness on the part of interpreters of what is required of them; this approach would require dedicated provision for audiology services alone.

A further problem noted with the use of interpreters was the tendency toward simplicity and filtering of information by professionals, while fuller information was provided to English-speaking parents. The use of family members as interpreters was regarded as distinctly unsatisfactory by some. At times, fathers were not perceived to be fully receptive to what they were being told, nor did they appear to share all the information with mothers. On the other hand, there were some perceived advantages in using family interpreters, such as being able to discuss the information when at home, and issues of confidentiality.

## Hearing aids and cochlear implants

Following diagnosis, parents and practitioners share common concerns about communication and language development. It was clear that parents held a range of views about hearing aids, cochlear implants, spoken and sign language and integrated as opposed to separate schooling. Here we discuss practitioners' views about hearing aids and cochlear implants.

Following diagnosis and the hearing aid recommendation, the provision of hearing aids was usually speedy, although commercial hearing aids could take longer than the recommended four weeks. Delays in the use of hearing aids by a child were exacerbated by the need to repeat the ear mould procedure and by missed appointments.

Purchasers regarded the satisfactory provision of aids as a fundamental priority. In one locality, the purchasers had ensured an enhanced budget for aids, to allow for increased purchase of commercial aids, while maintaining the existing levels of resource for cochlear implants. Some noted that although a hearing aid budget had always been identified, its split between support for children and adults was never clear.

In two of the localities there were no restrictions on providing commercial hearing aids. In another locality, however, practitioners and the local school for deaf children emphasised the need for more commercial aids which they regarded as more appropriate for some children. Access to commercial aids was restricted for children with moderate hearing loss and older children, although the more assertive parents were thought to be treated more favourably. The budget for aids in this locality had never been adequate and practitioners had not been presented with an opportunity to argue that the higher prevalence of deafness in their area meant they required more resources for aids than other areas with a similar population. This was exacerbated by children constituting a higher proportion of the deaf population requiring more back up resources for repairs and spares.

It was also suggested that health and education services could improve the link in the provision of aids. As a teacher noted:

> "... we hit a problem in that health, of course, only issue post-aural hearing aids, but the radio hearing aids are issued by education. So that link up becomes a little bit difficult at times, because while we're responsible for one area, and health are responsible for another, often a child is using one in conjunction with the other. So I'm not quite sure we've sort of linked that area up adequately either."

Opinions on the utility and appropriateness of *cochlear implants* differed. Some practitioners, particularly teachers, expressed concern about whether parents were coerced by consultants into accepting cochlear implants. This, they felt, did not offer parents an informed choice as advice was based on a definition of deafness as a tragic medical anomaly which could be corrected through technical interventions. A teacher stressed the need to consider the family's circumstances in making recommendations; she gave the example of a family with three deaf daughters where there was relatively good communication through signing and an acceptance of the Deaf culture and thus a cochlear implant was inappropriate.

In contrast, consultants generally regarded cochlear implants favourably. For some, deafness was a tragic disability which cochlear implants could put right; thus they found the reluctance of parents to opt for this service difficult to understand. They also felt justified in being assertive in their recommendations for implants because they firmly believed this to be in the child's best interests.

## Contracting and commissioning: 'a juggling act'

Purchasers' views on different aspects of services have been incorporated into the text. Here we discuss their perspectives on commissioning and means of ensuring effective and sensitive services for deaf children. A number of issues emerge.

Purchasers' views differed on the importance of needs assessment and epidemiological data in providing a more appropriate service. Among the problems cited were the changes in demography and inflow of both children and young adults into the locality. Many of these children may not be tested and many of the adults may not have been immunised. Women of childbearing age without rubella vaccination were mentioned specifically. It was generally agreed that 'prevention' can only ever remain a limited goal. Views on genetic counselling and consanguinity have been discussed elsewhere in these chapters. Purchasers noted that there were problems in screening programmes themselves, as discussed earlier with reference to other professionals.

Contracting remained a broad and imprecise activity, and some felt that it was not an effective vehicle for achieving change. To some purchasers, change required personal commitment and planning; the contracting process, through increased bureaucracy and short-termism, hampered medium to long-term planning. Contract specifications, being broadly defined, offered no solution to these difficulties. Purchasers also noted that purchasing services were as much about politics as about identified needs and there being demonstrably effective and cost-effective services to commission. Limited resources would always mean trade-offs between different services and different client groups. Priority setting was also influenced by individual whims and prejudices.

Even if certain priorities got written into contracts, the lack of specificity and problems in monitoring mean that accountability would remain limited. Purchasers argued that contracts are brief documents and can only set requirements at a general level, which does not allow detailed specifications or effective monitoring. Monitoring is hampered also by the aggregate nature of data collected by providers. And even when 'ethnic sensitivity' is specified, it is still left at a broad and vague level, such as emphasising language and communication needs.

## An ideal service

Despite some differences in scope and emphasis, there was common agreement that services needed to be *well coordinated*. This could be done by ensuring that a single *named person* had overall responsibility for the service, appointing *key workers* to ensure a coordinated service for parents, *improving links* between health and other agencies (eg, education), and a clearer role for social workers for deaf people. Practitioners were, however, keenly aware that most of their suggestions required extra resources in a climate where maintaining existing levels of funding was in itself a difficult task.

One suggestion made by a practitioner was that there should be a community paediatrician with a specialist interest in paediatric audiology who should coordinate services across the district, because if done piecemeal it would not be cost-effective. The person would need to have regard for other specialties and would collect, coordinate, and process information and pass it back to the other professionals involved. This person should also be responsible for auditing, research, setting up targets for the service, identifying pitfalls and rectifying problems. Appointment of a single senior person with a district-wide multidisciplinary team was also suggested by a respondent with senior level experience in social services:

> "... and there is a lot of mileage in experimenting with having education, health and social services and voluntary organisations working together with one person having strategic responsibility for that."

Such work would be jointly funded and well coordinated, avoiding the need for parents "to cope with a plethora of agencies that are around". A joint commissioning group could be responsible for overall purchasing, as noted by a senior social services respondent:

> "... I've argued for that in various places and attempted to try and get an authority to go down that line but not much success. If you went down that line, you can then get rid of this education/social services type split, put this amount of money into pre-five services and in order to do that we want to have three teachers of the deaf and a benefits advisor and an Asian worker or something like that and you can get rid of those distinctions [between different agencies]."

A practitioner in one of the localities suggested the idea of an easily accessible separate service for Asian families and drew on the example of provision of specialist services for Down's Syndrome children. However, both the advantages and disadvantages of this approach were appreciated. For example, a well coordinated and resourced service in one centre with all the specialties and language support while offering many advantages would exacerbate problems of physical access for many. A happy medium was difficult to achieve. In one locality, social services and the National Deaf Children's Society were working together to establish a 'one-stop' advocacy scheme so that parents could go to the advocacy service and someone could actually act as an advocate and try to cut through the system on their behalf. However, this was perceived to be both time and resource consumptive.

Stronger links between health and education services were also suggested as important. It would also be useful for parents to have a contact person with whom they could raise questions and queries by telephone. Use of this telephone service had not been possible previously because of the "services being split up and the parents being so confused as where to turn to". As far as dealing with social issues was concerned, feelings were expressed that the health visitors and teachers tended to perform the role of the social worker. Social services needed to be more centrally involved to facilitate a well coordinated and comprehensive service.

One consultant, who identified the main priority as being to increase the rate of attendance at appointments by Asian parents, stated there was a strong justification for employing a 'link worker' who could make home visits. This practitioner also stated that the link worker would not need to have extensive contact with other professionals. Their responsibility would be the identification of children at-risk and the need to ensure that they attended appointments. The link worker could also help in explaining to parents the cause of the deafness and inform them of support services. The last point is in contrast to views expressed by other practitioners that explanation about causation should be given by the consultant who discloses the diagnosis, followed up with detailed information and support by the teacher.

Within education, as well as health and social services, there was an appeal for more bilingual support and Asian workers who could provide language support, and more proactive, preventative work with families. There was a perceived need for greater cultural awareness on the part of the services. One suggestion was for a series of information booklets about the ethnic, cultural and religious proprieties of Asian users.

In one of the localities, the need for appropriate services was much more basic. This area relied on neighbouring localities for provision for deaf children. Practitioners, not surprisingly, felt that a locally-organised service would be very much appreciated by parents.

The legislative basis for fuller involvement of social services was emphasised by a senior social services respondent. The 1986 Disabled Persons Act places a duty on social services to collaborate with the local authority to plan the transfer of children with 'special needs' or disabilities into adulthood. The need for transitional plans is also mentioned in the 1981 Education Act. According to an experienced social service respondent:

> ".. certainly any child who has got a statement, there ought to be for each one of those a transitional plan, which sets out clearly the contribution ... that social services is going to make to that child's development from being a child into adulthood and what support they might need when they're in further education or getting work or how ... they access interpreting support, what sort of environmental support's going to be available, etc."

The 1989 Children Act also highlights the responsibilities of social services departments to coordinate services for children in need. These requirements, however, did not make social services a dominant or key player in service provision to these pre-school children; it may be that their role becomes more central for older deaf children. However, to provide for the wider needs of the deaf child and their family for social, emotional, financial and practical (eg, equipment) support, it is important to enhance the social services involvement in provision for young deaf children.

## Summary

This chapter has explored professionals' views about improving services. A number of suggestions were made to improve access to services. These included improvements in information to parents, more sympathetic disclosure with follow-up contact from the teacher, better coordination of services within and between agencies, and improved interpretation and translation provision. In terms of amplification support, improved collaboration between health and education services, and allocation of resources which takes account of the demographic and epidemiological profile rather than just the size of local population were regarded as important aspects of an improved service. There were differences between consultants and teachers about the utility of cochlear implants. Most consultants wished to see increased take-up; many teachers feared that parents were ill-informed about cochlear implants and were coerced into accepting them. Purchasers shared many of the concerns of other professionals regarding service coordination, resources and training. However, they regarded the commissioning process to be too broad, imprecise, short-term and cumbersome to be an effective tool for change. In considering an 'ideal service', improved coordination within and between agencies, appointment of a named senior person for district-wide responsibility for services, use of 'key workers' and 'link workers', improved communication, patient-friendly information and bilingual staff were offered as key elements.

# SEVEN

# Discussion of research findings

This chapter summarises the main research findings and synthesises parents' and professionals' accounts. The literature which forms the broader context for these findings is vast although, as noted, specific research on ethnicity and deafness remains limited and patchy; for brevity we make only limited reference to other studies. Of necessity the discussion of findings is brief; a fuller treatment of issues is available in the preceding chapters. For ease of presentation, we provide recommendations separately (Chapter 8).

## Legal and policy framework

Services for young deaf and disabled children require close working between health, social services, education and the voluntary sector. As Beresford et al (1996) note, recent policy legislation – for example, the 1989 Children Act; 1990 NHS and Community Care Act; 1993 Education Act; 1995 Children (Scotland) Act; 1995 Carers' (Support and Recognition) Act – demands a reconsideration of services provided to disabled children and their families. The 1997 Green Paper on special education entitled *Excellence for all children* emphasises the importance of regional planning for children with low incidence disabilities. This emerging policy could be particularly useful in harnessing scarce resources across an area, or between localities. Beresford et al (1996) note two positive changes in particular in this legislation and guidance. First, "obtaining the views of both parents and children has been acknowledged as a vital part of service provision, delivery and evaluation" (p 2). Second, they suggest that "the new market structures operating within health and social services have the capacity to promote innovation especially, perhaps, within the voluntary sector" (p 2). In considering the findings, the scope for innovation and the importance of parental views should be borne in mind.

## First suspicions and contact with health professionals

Early suspicions of deafness varied between parents. In families with a previous history of deafness, both the parents and professionals were vigilant and diagnoses were reached quickly. For most other children, a range of factors, such as the child's poor speech development, led to initial contact with health professionals. However, deafness was sometimes mistaken by parents for 'stubbornness' on the part of the child. For many children, hearing loss was picked up at routine developmental tests.

The health visitors played an important part in parents' contact with services and were valued by parents, although some parents felt that their concerns were not always taken seriously; a criticism they also levelled against GPs. The importance of parental views is increasingly recognised in services for disabled children (Beresford, 1995; Beresford et al, 1996). Parents, though sympathetic to the difficulties of diagnosing deafness, were critical that distraction tests sometimes failed to identify hearing loss. Parents felt that this lead to delays in diagnosis and had consequences for adjustment and appropriate support. Parents had relatively little contact with GPs, and felt them to be poorly informed about deafness.

## Screening and distraction tests

A number of issues were raised in relation to screening and distraction tests. The lack of nationally-agreed protocols for neonatal screening led to different policies; a problem noted also in relation to services for sickle cell disorders and thalassaemia (Atkin et al, 1998). Universal screening was not seen to be cost-effective. Professionals felt that technical as well as other problems (population inflow) meant that no screening programme could be effective in identifying all deaf children. Some of the localities had established selective screening through 'at-risk' registers to help identify families with a history of deafness; these facilitated earlier diagnosis than would otherwise be possible. Such selective screening also lacked standard protocols. Practitioners felt that the combination of the at-risk register, distraction tests and parental vigilance ensured the vast majority of deaf children were identified, although the potential for even earlier identification for a greater number of children may be there. One problem some professionals identified was that with the emphasis on 'at-risk' children and families, those deemed to be at 'low–risk' may not be identified sufficiently quickly. Greater benefits could be achieved by utilising existing screening systems more effectively, rather than introducing additional tests, and agreeing standard protocols. However, a recent major evaluation commissioned by the NHS with the involvement of the DoH and the National Deaf Children's Society is highly critical of selective screening, and deficiencies in the use of distraction tests (noted below). The authors recommended universal neonatal screening (Davis et al, 1997).

Distraction tests were felt by purchasers and providers to be a vital part of the service. Issues raised concerned the physical environment in which tests are performed, the importance of language in identifying the child's speech development, and training and skills required by health visitors. Distraction tests were often conducted under difficult circumstances: in rooms without sound proofing, often in the presence of siblings. Secondly, health visitors emphasised the social aspects of testing: talking to parents about the child, knowing the child and building rapport, having good interpersonal skills, taking history, and knowing about the child's first language. Not knowing relevant Asian languages, some felt, hampered successful testing (as in mispronouncing a child's name), especially in testing older children. Researchers and practitioners in other areas have also recognised this problem; one interesting response is the development of a Bengali language toy test for use in distraction tests (Bellman and Marcusson, 1991). Some felt that professionals often hold low expectations of disadvantaged and minority ethnic people in terms of language development; this may hinder the early identification of deafness. Finally, health visitors as well as other professionals felt that appropriate training, especially refresher courses for health visitors, was necessary. Many of these problems are highlighted by Davis et al (1997) and Ahmad et al (1998) discuss issues in training of staff working in the field of ethnicity and deafness more broadly.

Views differed on the possibility that Asian children may be being diagnosed later than white children. Most practitioners felt that at-risk registers and improved coordination of services had facilitated earlier diagnosis. Many believed that the age of fitting hearing aids had been brought down appreciably through these changes.

For various reasons, however, some professionals felt that Asian children may be being diagnosed later than white children. Missed appointments, prolonged visits to Pakistan, health visitors' less than optimal expertise with distraction tests, language barriers and not taking parents' concerns seriously were suggested as reasons. Problems of access to services for disabled children, as well as the importance of recognising parents' expertise in relation to their own children, have been emphasised in a number of recent publications (eg, Beresford, 1995; Beresford et al, 1996; Atkin et al, in press).

# Hearing aids and cochlear implants

Hearing aids and cochlear implants represent the main forms of technical support to deaf children. We discuss parents' and professionals' accounts about these.

## Hearing aids

On the whole, parents were satisfied, although some tensions and worries were noted. Parents' approach to the hearing aid use was often at variance with professional advice. Parents modified hearing aid use in a way which made sense to them, a finding also supported by other researchers (Fletcher, 1987; Robinson, 1991; see also Cartwright and Anderson, 1981; Hill, 1994). Both parents and children required time to adjust to using aids. Adjustment was influenced by a number of factors. Hearing aids which were relatively unobtrusive and less cumbersome were preferred, especially for very young children. Parents mentioned stigma, as well as victimisation in schools as some of the reasons for wanting aids which were more discrete. Many parents felt that they were better judges of how to use the aids and hence modification in length of time for which aids were to be worn seemed to them to be a perfectly logical response (see Beresford, 1995, for a broader discussion of 'parents as experts').

Practitioners felt that unique local demographic and epidemiological factors – in the case of West Yorkshire, for example, a high proportion of the Asian population who are perceived to be at greater risk of deafness – were not taken into account in setting budgets for amplification support. The service was thus under-resourced although it may have an appropriate allocation in terms of population size. Lack of clear division in the budgets, in terms of support for children and adults, was also problematic. Policies on commercial hearing aids differed. While most authorities allowed purchase of commercial aids, some placed restrictions on their purchase. The provision of aids was not well integrated between health services and education services in some of the localities. Joint purchasing mechanisms may help solve this problem to some extent.

## Cochlear implants

In this and related research (Ahmad et al, 1998), we have come across assumptions that Asian people prefer medical or technical solutions to health and other issues. A favourable view of cochlear implants would be consistent with this assumption. In fact, we found little enthusiasm for implants: parents were either against implants or remained ambivalent, views consistent with those of white parents more generally. Some had been told that implants were inappropriate for their children; these parents were less well informed about implants. However, parents of children for whom cochlear implants were appropriate were better informed, and had discussed the issue with family and professionals. For many, peripatetic teachers were the main source of information. Main points of concern were as follows. Parents remained to be convinced about the effectiveness of implants; some knew of cases where implants had not improved hearing to an extent that they felt justified the pain and discomfort of the procedure. As Hill (1994) notes, parents assess medical advice in the light of personal knowledge, and examples of perceived medical failures are often used to support personal judgements and resist medical advice (see also Atkin et al, in press). Finally, some were concerned about the perceived permanence of the procedure. Many parents saw this not in terms of a solution but as lasting damage to the child.

Practitioners were divided about cochlear implants. For example, a consultant was critical of parents who did not opt for implants; the practitioner's perspective being that deafness was a major deficit which could be rectified by implants. This practitioner questioned the parental right to refuse such treatment on behalf of the child. On the other hand, many practitioners, particularly peripatetic teachers, felt parents were unduly pressurised into accepting implants. This was seen as unethical, particularly as it occurred when parents were at their most vulnerable, soon after the diagnosis, and when they were not in a position to make an informed decision (see Atkin and Ahmad, 1998, for a broader discussion of ethical issues in service provision for disabilities).

## Causation and genetic counselling

Parents offered various causes for their child's deafness: asphyxia, complications during the baby's stay in intensive care, and other illnesses. Some did not have a clear idea of causation. However, many understood the primary cause to be parental consanguinity. Responses to consanguinity as a potential factor varied. Some expressed disbelief about its validity as it did not accord with their observation: why was it that some children were hearing and others deaf, why was there greater deafness in some consanguineous families than in others? Nor did parents always link consanguinity to genetics, a finding consistent with the work of Atkin et al (in press) and Atkin and Ahmad (1998). Atkin and Ahmad argue that genetic concepts occupy a realm which is distinct from that of lay understanding of inheritance and aetiology, a problem also shared by the white population. Some parents resented the attribution of deafness to consanguinity, which they felt undermined cherished practices. Such doubts about the validity of the consanguinity hypothesis discredit genetic counselling.

Professionals held differing views on the utility of genetic counselling; genetic counselling was a well-established regional resource with practice and research expertise. There was no system for routine referral of 'at-risk' families; no professional had explicit responsibility for referral; and there was little consensus among purchasers, providers and managers about an appropriate referral system. This troubled various professionals. On the one hand, there was a belief among a small number of professionals that consanguinity was the predominant cause of deafness, and this cultural practice needed to be challenged through genetic counselling. Some, in a more reflexive approach, felt that genetic counselling can provide helpful information for parents to aid decisions. Others remained unconvinced about the utility of genetic counselling; its low predictive power meant that its utility to parents, purchasers and providers was limited. Whatever the merits of these different positions, it is clear that many parents are being denied access to genetic knowledge and information which they may find useful, while others are given simplistic explanations which provoke guilt and raise doubts among parents about the motives of practitioners. Ahmad et al (forthcoming) discuss these issues in detail.

## Communication and access

Parents identified several communication problems of which lack of fluency in English and thus a need for interpreters is one. Others included:

- perceived poor communication between different health professionals and between health professionals and parents;
- inadequate time spent with parents in consultations and poor or no explanation;

- primary care professionals being ill-informed about deafness and consequently of little direct help.

Many parents felt that even when given an opportunity to ask for information they did not always know what to ask. This made parents reliant on professionals for all relevant information and supported the belief that "professionals know what we want" (see also Ahmad et al, 1998). Professionals, for their part, felt that Asian parents were not sufficiently assertive in seeking information.

Face-to-face communication remained a problem for one third of these relatively young parents. Using spouses, family or friends as interpreters was common. This was taken for granted so that none of the parents without skills in English expressed overt concerns about the relative lack of interpreting provision.

Although not mentioned as a particular problem by parents, poor interpreting services and other problems of communication caused major concerns to practitioners as well as purchasers. That there is bad practice is confirmed by practitioners – peripatetic teachers and health visitors in particular. No locality had a dedicated interpreting service. Most relied on the often overstretched hospital-wide service. Even when interpreters were available there were problems. One problem concerned the speed with which interpreting support could be summoned. Some practitioners, with justification, were critical of using family members for interpreting (see Shackman, 1985; Askham et al, 1995; Ahmad and Walker, 1997).

The second problem concerned the lack of training of interpreters as well as the professionals who used interpreters. Professionals felt that inappropriate filtering on the part of themselves as well as interpreters occurred routinely, and that parents who did not need an interpreter received fuller and more contextual information. Thirdly, some practitioners raised the issue of sensitivity and empathy; they felt that a service which was integral to audiology would share a common ethos, have a positive rapport with other colleagues and would be of greater value. Ahmad et al (1998) discuss many related issues in relation to ethnicity and deafness. Problems of generic interpreters and using unqualified interpreters in the area of ethnicity and deafness are discussed by Ahmad et al (1998) and more generally by Shackman (1985) and the Health Education Authority (1997).

Professionals also discussed the role of information and other aspects of access to services.

## Information

Professionals felt that Asian families remained poorly served in terms of information. Language barriers, poor interpreting facilities, few bilingual staff and limited translated materials, all contributed to an information vacuum. Consequently, parents coped and made decisions with insufficient knowledge and support. This is a problem which particularly confronts mothers. Literature suggests that mothers are generally more knowledgeable about a child's condition than fathers; this greater information equips them to deal with the day-to-day physical, emotional and social care of the child (Ahmad and Atkin, 1996a). However, the evidence from our study as well as by Atkin et al (in press) suggests that Asian women tend to be particularly poorly informed about the child's condition and sources of help, and that the information gap is not adequately filled by increased input from fathers.

## Disclosure

Appropriate disclosure is regarded as vital for parental adjustment and ensuring adequate support and information (Sloper and Turner, 1992; for a review see Beresford et al, 1996). Many practitioners felt that the diagnosis was poorly explained and the physical environment was rarely conducive to sensitive handling of parents' concerns and emotions. Discussions about disclosure often took place in a room with numerous people waiting outside for their turn. Where peripatetic teachers were involved, explanations were sometimes offered in the hospital corridor. A more conducive environment offering privacy would facilitate improved disclosure and information exchange. Practitioners also felt that there was a lack of clarity between the roles of the consultant and the peripatetic teacher; some felt that the consultant should offer fuller explanation while others felt this was best done by the peripatetic teacher.

On the whole, parents felt that the diagnosis was disclosed appropriately. Disclosure which was sympathetic and sensitive, where sufficient time was given to parents and where parents were allowed or encouraged to ask questions, was much appreciated. Parents disliked disclosure in a mechanistic, unsympathetic or rushed style. Sloper and Turner (1992), in relation to children with disabilities more generally, note that parents valued a sympathetic manner, and understanding of their concerns and an opportunity for further questions after the disclosure. Fletcher (1987) and Robinson (1991) both write of the importance of the manner in which the diagnosis is given of a child's deafness.

However, information exchange during the diagnostic consultation remained problematic. Parents wanted information on aetiology, prognosis and implications of deafness for themselves and the child. One area of concern was that the consultants should provide more information and encourage parents to return to seek clarifications; parents had to rely on peripatetic teachers for such information, and although generally satisfied with peripatetic teachers, for some parents the lack of information from consultants remained an issue. Second, for some the information could have come earlier; the time lag between disclosure and meeting with the peripatetic teacher was sometimes considered too long and exacerbated parental worries. Other research shows that parents require consolidation of new knowledge through access to information on an ongoing basis and such information must address the changing needs as the child develops and moves through services – the ongoing contact with consultants or peripatetic teachers may usefully serve this function (Baldwin and Carlisle, 1994; Beresford et al, 1996; Ahmad et al, 1998).

## Improving attendance at appointments

Many parents had problems with the appointments system: long delays between appointments; late referrals; unhelpful receptionists; delays in seeing professionals despite being given a specific appointment time; and too short a time with the professional. In particular, those with two or more deaf children found it difficult to juggle appointments in different departments for different children. Some parents felt that professionals informed them of the appointment too far in advance with no reminders closer to the date. Finally, the perceived inflexibility of appointments, coupled with the lack of interpreting facilities, often meant that the working father took unpaid leave to attend the appointment. Weekend access for audiological equipment and repairs was suggested as something that would be helpful. Research shows a generally positive attitude towards child health services by Asian parents (Baker et al, 1984; Watson, 1984; Kurtz, 1993) and therefore the problems of non-attendance are unlikely to be due entirely to parental apathy.

Professionals felt that attendance at appointments was poor; reasons for this were contested. A minority, including some purchasers, felt Asian parents were particularly poor at keeping appointments. Visits abroad, presumed lack of concern about children and a suspicion that appointments for girls were less likely to be attended than for boys were offered as reasons. Some also felt that Asian parents have greater expectations of external help, such as transport, to attend appointments.

However, a majority blamed administrative, personal and environmental barriers for missed appointments; views consistent with parental accounts. Childcare was one such barrier – parents often had to juggle appointments between different clinics and even different provider trusts. Appointments rarely took into account childcare responsibilities, resulting in siblings accompanying the deaf child and thus having their education disrupted, or the parent missing the appointment. Transport posed clear difficulties, as also noted in parents' accounts – use of public transport was made difficult by language problems, travel distances and accompanying children. Appointments were often changed at very short notice. Long waits and inadequate time with the consultant led to parents questioning the value of the consultation. As a purchaser noted, some of these problems result from the block booking system in many of the clinics. Many practitioners felt that improved administration could solve some of these problems.

## Reactions to diagnosis

Parents responded to diagnoses in a variety of ways. For most, it was a traumatic experience which required time for adjustment. (Our sample, however, was made up predominantly of hearing parents; quite different responses may be found among parents who are deaf themselves.) Reactions, including disbelief, denial, anger, grief, and feelings of divine punishment, are consistent with those reported by others in relation to childhood disability (Baldwin and Carlisle, 1994; Beresford et al, 1996; Atkin et al, in press). The little contact with social services may result in a relative lack of emotional support for parents. Some social workers with the deaf felt that there was a clear role for them in providing support to parents, but in practice this was impeded by a lack of clarity in professional division of labour and poor interagency collaboration.

Some parents disagreed with the diagnosis. Parents and families also used a variety of discourses to sustain 'denial', including personal observations which some felt were inconsistent with diagnosis, comparing the child with hearing children, and for one father, a scientist, the lack of 'scientific evidence' for the diagnosis (see Hill, 1994 and Atkin and Ahmad, in press, in relation to haemoglobin disorders).

Parents' views on the time taken to reach diagnosis varied. On the whole, parents were sympathetic to the problems of reaching diagnosis quickly and took account both of human fallibility and the crudeness of techniques. Problems remained, however. As noted, some were unhappy that their views are not taken seriously by health visitors, GPs and other professionals. Others expressed incredulity that the distraction tests do not pick up deafness and had questions about whether these tests were being applied appropriately. Finally, there were concerns about not knowing the time of onset of deafness; this concerned particularly those parents whose children were not diagnosed quickly. Many of these concerns echo those expressed by parents of children with other conditions, such as sickle cell disorder or thalassaemia (Hill, 1994; Atkin et al, in press) as well as parents with deaf children (Fletcher, 1987; Robinson, 1991; and Gregory, 1973).

The reactions of the wider family follow similar patterns, not surprising considering that parents' own reactions are influenced by discussions with family, friends and professionals (see also Hill, 1994).

## Family support and caring

Wider family involvement with deaf children and their parents shows many parallels with what is reported in research studies on caring (Twigg, 1992; Baldwin and Carlisle, 1994; Twigg and Atkin, 1994). The family constituted a valued and flexible resource; those without close kin living nearby missed such support. Most had close kin nearby on whom they relied for both emotional and practical support (for wider debates, see Anwar, 1979; Warrier, 1988; Twigg, 1992; Ahmad, 1996b). However, not all found the family supportive. Parents were highly ambivalent about some forms of 'help', such as 'compensatory' attention which 'spoilt' the deaf child. Consistent with the wider literature (Ahmad and Atkin, 1996a; 1996b), both the 'caring about' and 'caring for' tasks were generally confined to parents, mainly mothers.

Caring had both pleasurable, and routine and mundane aspects (see Twigg, 1992; Ahmad and Atkin, 1996a; 1996b). Mothers dealt with routine caring. Some parents felt having a deaf child affected their employment, and carried additional costs, such as for environmental aids (see Baldwin and Carlisle, 1994, for more general review). Communication posed problems and made caring for a deaf child more difficult than for a hearing child. Learning extra skills, such as BSL, and liaison with the school for deaf children were regarded as important, but additional tasks, with time, cost and social implications. Some parents expressed concerns about the future; a commonly noted feature of the caring literature (eg, Ahmad and Atkin, 1996a; 1996b). They were worried about the child, educationally and socially, feeling that the child will have lifelong needs for parental support. However, like all parents, these parents also found considerable enjoyment in caring for their deaf children. This related to pleasure in children's achievements and their endearing qualities.

## Religion and culture

Ideas about religion were intermeshed with rituals, beliefs, lifestyles, gendered roles, cultural values and social life (see Ahmed, 1989). In talking about the importance of religion to deaf children, parents emphasised the social aspects of religious life, such as gender roles and age and gender appropriate behaviour rather than rituals. Ahmad et al (1998) report a range of activity led by minority ethnic deaf people and their families around religious and cultural identity. Parents expressed concerns about instilling appropriate cultural values in their deaf children; as Ahmad et al (1998) argue, this may have particular salience for parents of deaf children who experience greater difficulty in their children's religious and cultural socialisation, a process in which spoken language plays a large part in hearing families.

Religion was also important in helping parents make sense of the child's deafness. Parents often made references to 'God's will' and 'destiny' in talking about deafness. However, we found little evidence of complacency. Consistent with Atkin and Ahmad's (in press) findings in relation to parents caring for children with thalassaemia, parental belief in destiny was coupled with a sense of responsibility to do the best for their child.

## Knowledge and perceptions of deafness

Little is written about attitudes to deafness or disability within the Asian communities (but see Abedi, 1988; Stuart 1992; Miles, 1993; Begum et al, 1994). Knowledge of and attitudes to deafness, deaf culture and sign language varied between parents. Some were knowledgeable and motivated to learn more about these issues. Many felt that deafness was negatively perceived and that this was consistent with the disablism in the Asian and white communities (see also Ahmad et al, 1998). On the whole, parents' limited knowledge of deafness is consistent with low levels of knowledge of other conditions affecting children (Ahmad and Atkin, 1996a; Atkin et al, in press). This has implications for services. For optimum care, parents need to know about the child's condition and relevant services; without adequate information, parents often cope without appropriate service support (see Chamba et al, forthcoming: a).

## Language and communication choice for children

Gregory et al (1995) found in their study of deaf young people that "where families had learnt to sign this had facilitated communication and most felt they should have been offered information and advice about sign language from the start". Alongside this, the spoken languages other than English are also important. Ahmad et al (1998) note that much of the user-led activity by minority ethnic deaf people centres around issues of cultural identity. Access to community language is a major vehicle for gaining full community membership and cultivating an ethnic identity which may have influenced language choices made by parents of deaf children who opt for spoken languages rather than sign language.

Attitudes to language choice and communication strategies varied among parents. Influencing factors included the degree of the child's deafness, parental preferences, previous experiences, available support, professional advice and concerns about education and integration in the deaf and/or ethnic community. Some showed prejudice against sign language and/or felt influenced by perceived societal prejudice against signing. Parents showed greater support for spoken language development than for sign language.

On the whole, parents were influenced by professional advice (largely from peripatetic teachers) which varied between: home language ('to help cultural identity development'); sign language ('to facilitate language development'); English only ('to avoid confusion'); and a variety of languages, both spoken and sign. Discussions with peripatetic teachers confirmed this and variation was as much a reflection of peripatetic teachers' personal philosophy and local policy as it was due to the degree of hearing loss or family characteristics and preferences (for more detail, see Chamba et al, forthcoming: b). On the whole, parents used a variety of languages with children with an increasing use of home language. However, some parents remained confused about language choice; a confusion fuelled also by their uncertainty about the degree of the child's deafness. Ahmad et al (1998) report that families of deaf people felt that there had been a welcome change in peripatetic teachers' approaches to community languages, a view confirmed by peripatetic teachers in this study. Consistent with Ahmad et al, some parents felt that unquestioning acceptance of professional advice to use only English with deaf children undermined the child's sense of cultural identity and compromised communication with the wider family (see also Gregory et al, 1995; Ahmad et al, 1998). This was perceived to have had long-term implications for older deaf children whose parents had been advised in this way (see Chamba et al, forthcoming: b).

Many mothers were learning BSL or sign supported English (see also Ahmad et al, 1998, for a national perspective). Very few fathers made an effort to learn sign language. In addition to learning signing, parents also valued the social aspects of such classes; an important resource in terms of information, practical help and social support, as noted also by Ahmad et al (1998). Parents were poorly informed about the bilingual education debate.

Language and communication choice is a complex issue for parents and professionals alike. There is little knowledge about how BSL is used in conjunction with English and other spoken languages. Although in some areas, families and some teachers have developed ways of using different languages, this knowledge remains localised and is not written about (Susan Gregory, personal communication, 1998).

## Commissioners' perspectives

Commissioning offers opportunities to influence the shape and scope of services for children. Beresford et al (1996) note, in particular, the scope for encouraging interagency working and collaboration. We have integrated purchasers' perspectives throughout the text. Here we discuss views on commissioning as a tool for improving services. Purchasers felt that need assessment and demographic profiling were of limited help in identifying specific needs and that the purchasing mechanisms worked at too broad a level to allow close monitoring or evaluation. Even if needs could be clearly identified, itself a difficult task, priority setting was a politically fraught activity. Some felt that within the politics of 'juggling priorities', ethnicity did not have a high status.

It was also felt that even when 'ethnic sensitivity' is specified, it is at a broad level; detail is worked out by the trust. The monitoring data provided by the trusts are about activity and costs, and not about quality and sensitivity. The ability of purchasers to effect change was thus limited. Change, some argued, depended on medium to long-term planning and commitment on the part of individuals within organisations. Flynn et al (1996) have studied the politics of purchasing and note some of the problems identified here.

## Collaboration and service coordination

The importance of interagency working in services for children with disabilities is stressed in recent legislation and research. Parents find professional and agency boundaries puzzling. Poor collaboration also leads to uncertainties over areas of responsibility. These issues are summarised here.

Not surprisingly, parents found the demarcation between the role of different agencies puzzling and unhelpful. For parents, issues of language choice and caring, housing, resources, equipment and costs were all intertwined and difficult to compartmentalise into needs which neatly fitted the remit of particular agencies (see Glendinning, 1985).

Access to sign language teaching and information on deafness and Deaf culture was facilitated largely by peripatetic teachers, who often assumed the role of 'key worker'. In addition to information and practical help, most parents also found contact with the school for deaf children helpful: practical support as well as social contact with other children and parents were valued. Ahmad et al (1998) report that parents expressed a need for a variety of information and support – information about deafness, advice on benefits, meeting deaf adults, access to sign language, practical help with forms and welfare rights, skills and assertiveness to deal with powerful professionals, and emotional support.

Although valuing peripatetic teachers, parents did not follow their advice uncritically; nor did peripatetic teachers have homogenous views (note variation in advice on language choice above; see also Chamba et al, forthcoming: b). Decisions were often finely balanced, and as in language choice, the child's characteristics, personal preferences and appropriate resources in schools were all important considerations. Parents saw both the costs and benefits of mainstream schools and schools for deaf children. However, many were pleasantly surprised by the educational achievements of deaf children at schools for deaf children. And those who had opted for a mainstream school gave serious thought to the level and appropriateness of support for deaf children, as well as the potential reaction of hearing children. Many of these concerns are shared by families of deaf children generally (eg, Gregory et al, 1995; Ahmad et al, 1998). Some were relieved that the local schools for deaf children now included instruction on minority cultures and religions. Ahmad et al (1998, ch 5) note the lack of such instruction, and the white Christian ethos of such schools being of concern both to deaf young people and their families, succinctly put by a mother: "I send my child to school and he comes back an Englishman".

The lack of social services involvement, where it was felt to be needed by parents, was worrying. Very few parents had any contact with social services. Social services have an important potential role to play, ranging from the emotional support of parents, and advice on benefits, to provision of equipment and adaptations. Those who were in contact with social services valued the practical support with benefits and dealings with housing and other departments. The importance of such practical support is clear in research literature (Beresford et al, 1996). The absence of social services' involvement is surprising considering the emphasis on the role of social services for provision to disabled children in recent legislation and policy guidance. Although social services were involved in the Centres for the Deaf, their role in services for young deaf children remained marginal in all study sites. However, Ahmad et al (1998) note that nationally, social services are responsible for supporting many initiatives on ethnicity and deafness with deaf adults (see Darr et al, 1997, for examples of initiatives).

There was little use of voluntary organisations. Few parents knew about such help or used voluntary organisations. However, it may be that relatively little of this activity focuses on pre-school deaf children. Ahmad et al (1998) report criticism of the deaf organisations by minority ethnic deaf people and their families; deaf organisations were often seen to marginalise issues of ethnicity, to be doing little to counter racism among workers and white members and having little representation from minority ethnic deaf people or their families among workers and management committees. More positively, they also note improvements in some Deaf voluntary organisations.

Problems of coordination also hampered smooth collaborative work between different professionals within the same agency. Often services were split between separate hospitals within the same provider trust, leading to redundancy and duplication, and confusion on the part of parents who may be requested to attend different hospitals for different procedures, or for different children. Communication remained poor between health visitors and secondary care; health visitors felt that their role would become more effective if they were routinely informed about children's progress through the system. GPs remained marginal to services for deaf children.

## An ideal service

Professionals' perspectives on an 'ideal service' for Asian deaf children stressed a number of issues; many of these have been discussed earlier:

- a single senior person with the responsibility for the whole service to ensure inter- and intra-agency integration, and with an overall dedicated budget (see SMAC Report, 1994 for similar recommendations for haemoglobinopathy services);

- a 'key worker' approach to parental support to ensure coordinated services;
- improved collaborative links between health and education as well as between health and social services, and the voluntary sector;
- integrated provision through comprehensive centres offering the full range of facilities covering the remit of health, education and social services;
- improvements in appointment systems through better language support, closer liaison between consultants and booking clerks and outreach work;
- improved screening through better use of screening procedures, training of health visitors and other staff and smaller caseloads to ensure more 'quality time' with children and parents.

Parents' views on improving services are integrated in the discussion. Here we note their specific advice to other parents. Perhaps most importantly, many suggested the need for early referral. The importance of early diagnosis was recognised by most parents; they felt that parents should trust personal judgement and be assertive in their dealings with professionals. That parents are experts on their own children is increasingly being recognised (Beresford, 1995; Beresford et al, 1996); although as noted, many parents felt that their views were not taken seriously by professionals, an issue noted by Atkin and Ahmad (in press) in relation to interaction between parents of children with haemoglobin disorders and professionals. Parents felt that extra vigilance is required to ensure the safety of a deaf child, ranging from care in the home to crossing roads. Finally, some felt it important to value sign language and to act quickly to learn it. The importance of effective communication with the child was emphasised and perceived to have long-term implications. Parents also wanted support with information to make informed decisions about language and education, caring and costs, and the provision of environmental and hearing aids.

## Conclusion

Two common problems plague research on ethnicity and health (Ahmad, 1996a). One is that the difference between minority and majority ethnic populations is overemphasised and the far greater similarities between them are ignored. Second, the heterogeneity of backgrounds, views and experiences among the minority populations is underplayed. Both problems result in an approach which emphasises distinct and different needs at the level of broadly-defined ethnic groups. Instead, reality is more complex. As this study shows, there are many similarities in the experiences and views of Asian and white parents of deaf children; Asian parents of deaf children and Asian parents of children with other disabilities; and these Asian parents' interaction with services and the relationship of minority ethnic populations with the welfare state more generally. Herein lies both a problem and hope. The problem rests in not being able to provide a simple recipe dictating what 'specifically' and uniquely should be done to cater for the needs of Asian parents of deaf children. The many commonalities, as noted, make such a response untenable. The hope is in a recognition that an improved service which respects partnership with parents and recognises their expertise over their own children will also serve those from minority ethnic groups. For this, parents need to be appropriately informed about deafness and its implications, and provided with the necessary service support for the child and themselves. As parents' and professionals' accounts confirm, much progress needs to be made to achieve this simple goal.

# EIGHT

# Recommendations for improving services for Asian deaf children

Chapter 7 has summarised the key research findings and provided the research and policy context for their interpretation. Here we set out the key recommendations. For convenience, we note our recommendations under particular headings: legislation, service organisation, screening, access and information, diagnosis and disclosure, hearing aids and cochlear implants, culture and language choice, and interprofessional and interagency working. Clearly, the recommendations need to be prioritised in line with local demographic and epidemiological profiles. The recommendations should be used as a basis for developing action plans for integrated children's services. As we note at the end of Chapter 7, Asian parents' needs for information and support are not fundamentally different from those of other parents with deaf children. Many of the recommendations are therefore broad-based. However, those which have particular relevance to Asian parents have been *italicised*.

## Legislation

- *Purchasers and providers in the NHS, practitioners and policy makers in education, social services and the voluntary sector should ensure that services are culturally appropriate and be aware of the duties placed on them to provide support for 'children in need'. Services for Asian deaf children and families should be included in Children's Services Plans which are now mandatory.*

## Service organisation

- NHS purchasers should ensure that resources reflect local demographic profiles when agreeing budgets.

- *Systems for ethnic monitoring of service provision should be established with guidance from purchasers.*

- *Purchasers should work with providers to establish guidelines for ethnically-sensitive services. These may have generic features (interpreting support, food, etc) with some service specific elements. Parents groups and voluntary organisations could provide valuable advice on appropriate guidelines.*

- *Budgets for hearing aids should take into consideration the split between adult and child users and be weighted accordingly.*

- The demarcation between the role of health services and education services in hearing aid provision and maintenance should be examined to facilitate collaborative working.

- *The relative advantages and disadvantages of locally-based clinics offering easy access, and centrally-coordinated and comprehensive multiagency centres providing the range of services, including language support, required by parents of deaf children should be considered in setting up community services.*

## Screening

- There should be improved communication between different healthcare professionals (eg, GPs, health visitors and consultants) to facilitate a better service to parents of deaf children.

- *Improved screening should be implemented through better use of screening procedures including ongoing training of health visitors, and other staff, and allowing professionals more 'quality time' with Asian parents and their deaf children to improve detection rates.*

- Health and education professionals, in consultation with purchasers and other stakeholders, should develop protocols for testing and screening to provide maximum coverage of children.

- Registers containing information on families with a previous history of deafness facilitate early diagnosis of deafness. Providers and purchasers should consider establishing such registers, with agreed protocols for referrals and monitoring.

- Practitioners should ensure that distraction tests are conducted in a suitable environment by appropriately trained staff. This has been identified as a major problem in a national review (Davis et al, 1997).

- *Familiarity with the child's language is important in testing. If professionals, particularly health visitors, do not have familiarity with the child's or family's spoken language, employment of bilingual assistants, language training and use of appropriate materials (eg, word list in relevant languages) should be considered.*

- *Health and education professionals should establish if there are systematic differences in the age of diagnosis between Asian and other deaf children and the provision of appropriate amplification support and seek mechanisms to improve the speed with which these services are provided to Asian families.*

## Access and information

- *ENT and audiology practitioners should examine the appointments systems and seek means of enhancing attendance by Asian parents.*

- *Parents should be given accessible information about appointments and sent reminders closer to the time – this should include information on location, time, as well as purpose of the visit.*

- Parents should be given a time for their appointment and administrative staff and practitioners should ensure delays in seeing parents are kept to a minimum. Parents should be informed of reasons for unexpected delays.

- *Administrative staff should be culturally sensitive; staff whom parents regard as incompetent, rude or racist are unlikely to facilitate attendance.*

- Parents should be given flexibility in arranging appointments to allow for childcare and job-related contingencies.

- Administrative staff and practitioners should ensure that last minute changes in appointment dates, times and venues are avoided. Frequent changes lead to a lack of confidence in the service and will not enhance attendance.

- Consultations should allow enough time to address parental concerns.

- Information about possible genetic causes should be provided to parents. This should be done in a balanced and non-judgemental way.

- *Referral systems for genetic counselling should be established. Professionals should handle such referrals sensitively without victim or culture-blaming.*

- *Professionals should ensure that parents have accessible information in appropriate media (language, audio, video) about the diagnosis, likely causes of deafness, future prospects for the deaf child, and sources of support.*

- *Training needs of interpreters (both in Asian languages and BSL), and practitioners and administrative staff who work with interpreters should be addressed.*

- *Language needs of parents should be provided for, using trained interpreters, to ensure informed participation in their child's welfare. Purchasers and providers have a responsibility to provide a culturally-appropriate service; enabling parents to communicate with practitioners is a basic element of such a service.*

- *Using family members and friends for interpreting constitutes unacceptable and bad practice. This should be avoided.*

- *In areas with significant numbers of Asian users, a dedicated interpreting service should be instituted for audiology. This ensures that interpreters have relevant service knowledge, rapport between interpreters and the professionals who use them and continuity of service for parents.*

## Diagnosis and disclosure

- *Parental concerns about the child's hearing are important in identifying childhood deafness and should be taken seriously by professionals.*

- *Parents should be kept informed of the process of screening and testing. Difficulties in reaching diagnosis or making precise predictions about language development should be explained.*

- It is vital that the diagnosis is appropriately explained to parents, allowing an opportunity to gain information on causation and implications for the child's language development. Parents should be encouraged to return, if necessary, to ask questions at a later date.

- Sensitivity of approach is as important as perceived clinical competence. Practitioners should ensure disclosure takes place in a private room and is not hurried.

- Referrals to peripatetic teachers should be made to ensure parents are provided with necessary information and ongoing support soon after the diagnosis.

- Parents' needs for emotional support should be considered and addressed. This may be done by the peripatetic teacher and the consultant, but there is scope for social services and the voluntary sector to play an increasing role.

## Hearing aids and cochlear implants

- *Information and support should be given to parents about hearing aid use. Contact with other Asian parents whose children use aids and with deaf adults who used aids as children may be of help.*

- *Parents need balanced information, in appropriate languages or other media, about cochlear implants to make informed decisions.*

- Parental concerns and difficulties about hearing aid use – child's discomfort, obtrusiveness, fears of bullying – should be addressed by professionals.

## Culture and language choice

- *The wider Asian family constitutes a flexible and valued resource whose needs for information and influences on parents should be respected by professionals.*

- *Not all Asian parents have access to a supportive extended family. Professionals should avoid stereotyped assumptions about familial support and be aware of individual parental needs for social, practical and emotional support.*

- *Parents' concerns about passing on appropriate religious and cultural values to their deaf children and about their children's development of a positive cultural identity should be addressed.*

- *Access to home language is an important part of developing cultural identity and, where appropriate, professionals should seriously consider providing support to children for development of home language.*

- *Parents should be provided with information and support to make informed decisions about language choice for their deaf children.*

- *Provision of speech and language therapy in relevant Asian languages should be considered where the child is learning spoken languages.*

- *To facilitate greater understanding of deafness, parents should be given access to balanced information in appropriate languages and to positive deaf role models from their own communities.*

- *The importance of sign language learning should be emphasised to parents and access to sign language learning should be improved. In particular, efforts should be made to recruit more fathers into sign language classes. Professionals should explore the possibility of encouraging sign language learning at home.*

- *Education services, in consultation with health services, the deaf voluntary sector and parents' groups, should agree a broad policy on language and communication, including support for home language development. This should minimise inconsistencies in advice to parents on language and communication from different staff.*

## Interprofessional and interagency working

- Close interagency collaboration, especially between the health and education service, but with the involvement of social services and the deaf voluntary sector, should be developed to ensure a coordinated and coherent service to Asian parents.

- Collaboration between services for disabled children under five years of age suggests good models of practice. However, collaboration between health and social services, and health and the voluntary sector, remains poor for provision to pre-school deaf children. The potential role of other agencies should be carefully considered by NHS purchasers and providers and good working relationships should be cultivated.

- Clear and effective communication channels between professionals involved should be established both within the hospital sector, and between hospital and community health and primary care services.

- *Communication systems between professionals and parents should be developed to ensure parents have access to relevant information at the right time, and know where to seek information when required.*

- *Parents find demarcation between the remit of different agencies puzzling and unhelpful. Allocation of professionals (such as peripatetic teachers) with a 'key worker' role who provide information and help coordinate services between different agencies to work with Asian families should be considered.*

- The possible enhanced role of social services in providing guidance on benefits and environmental aids, as well as emotional support to parents should be considered.

- *The deaf voluntary sector which deals with deaf children and their parents should carefully examine their role in relation to Asian parents and enhance support to these parents.*

- A single person with an overall dedicated budget and responsibility for the whole service to ensure inter- and intra-agency collaboration would facilitate a coordinated service for deaf children. Services should consider the potential for pooling budgets.

# References and further reading

Abedi, R. (1988) *From sound to silence,* London: Hobo.

Ahmad, W.I.U. (ed) (1993) *'Race' and health in contemporary Britain,* Buckingham: Open University Press.

Ahmad, W.I.U. (1994) 'Reflections on the consanguinity and birth outcome debate', *Journal of Public Health Medicine,* vol 16, no 4, pp 423-8.

Ahmad, W.I.U. (1996a) 'The trouble with culture', in D. Kelleher and S. Hillier (eds) *Researching cultural differences in health,* London: Routledge.

Ahmad, W.I.U. (1996b) 'Family obligations and social change among Asian communities', in W.I.U. Ahmad and K. Atkin (eds) *'Race' and community care,* Buckingham: Open University Press.

Ahmad, W.I.U. and Atkin, K. (1996a) 'Ethnicity and childhood disability: the case of sickle cell disorder and thalassaemia', *British Journal of Social Work,* vol 26, pp 755-75.

Ahmad, W.I.U. and Atkin, K. (ed) (1996b) *'Race' and community care,* Buckingham: Open University Press.

Ahmad, W.I.U. and Walker, R. (1997) 'Health and social care needs of Asian older people', *Ageing and Society,* vol 17, pp 141-65.

Ahmad, W.I.U., Atkin, K. and Chamba, R. (forthcoming) '"Causing havoc among their children": parents' and professionals perspectives on consanguinity and childhood disability', *Sociology of Health and Illness.*

Ahmad, W.I.U., Darr, A. and Jones, L. (in press) "I send my child to school and he comes back an Englishman": Minority ethnic deaf people, identity politics and services', in W.I.U. Ahmad (ed) *Ethnicity, disability and caring,* Buckingham: Open University Press.

Ahmad, W.I.U., Darr, A., Jones, L. and Nisar, G. (1998) *Deafness and ethnicity: Services, policy and politics,* Bristol: The Policy Press.

Ahmed, A.S. (1989) *Discovering Islam,* London: Routledge.

Anionwu, E. (1993) 'Sickle cell and thalassaemia: community experiences and official response', in W.I.U. Ahmad (ed) *'Race' and health in contemporary Britain,* Buckingham: Open University Press.

Anwar, M. (1979) *The myth of return: Pakistanis in Britain*, London: Heinemann.

Askham, J., Henshaw, L. and Tarpey, M. (1995) *Social and health authority services for elderly people from black and ethnic minorities*, London: HMSO.

Atkin, K. and Ahmad, W.I.U. (1998) 'Genetic screening and haemoglobinopathies: ethics, politics and practice', *Social Science and Medicine*, vol 46, no 3, pp 445-58.

Atkin, K., Ahmad, W.I.U. and Anionwu, E.N. (1998) 'Service support to families caring for a child with a sickle cell disorder or thalassaemia: the experience of health professionals, service managers and health commissioners', *Health*, vol 2, no 3, pp 305-27.

Atkin, K., Ahmad, W.I.U. and Anionwu, E.N. (in press) 'Genetic screening for sickle cell disorder and thalassaemia: parents' and professionals' accounts', *Social Science and Medicine*.

Badat, H. and Whall-Roberts, D. (1994) *Bridging the gap: Creating services for deaf people from ethnic minority communities*, London: RNID.

Baker, M.R., Bandranayake, R. and Schweiger, M.S. (1984) 'Difference in rate of uptake of immunization among ethnic groups', *British Medical Journal*, vol 288, pp 1075-8.

Baldwin, S. and Carlisle, J. (1994) *Social support for disabled children and their families*, London: HMSO.

Begum, N., Hill, M. and Stevens, A. (1994) *Reflections: Views of black disabled people on their lives and community care*, London: Central Council for Education and Training in Social Work.

Bellman, S. and Marcusson, M. (1991) 'A new toy test to investigate hearing status of young children who have English as a second language', *British Journal of Audiology*, vol 25, pp 317-22.

Beresford, B. (1995) *Expert opinions: A survey of parents caring for a severely disabled child*, Bristol: The Policy Press.

Beresford, B., Sloper, T., Baldwin, S. and Newman, T. (1996) *What works in services for families with a disabled child*, Ilford: Barnardos.

Bhopal, R. and Samin, A.K. (1988) 'Immunization uptake of Glasgow Asian children', *Community Medicine*, vol 10, pp 215-20.

Cartwright, A. and Anderson, R. (1981) *General practice revisited*, London: Tavistock.

Chamba, R., Ahmad, W.I.U. and Hirst, M. (forthcoming: a) *Expert voices: A survey of minority ethnic families with disabled children*, Bristol: The Policy Press.

Chamba, R., Ahmad, W.I.U. and Jones, L. (forthcoming: b) 'Language, communication and cultural identity: perspectives on Asian deaf children', *Deafness and Education*.

Chamba, R., Ahmad, W.I.U., Darr, A. and Jones, L. (1998) 'Education of Asian deaf children', in S. Gregory, P. Knight, W. McCrackon, S. Powers and L. Watson (eds) *Education of deaf children*, London: David Fulton.

Christensen, K. and Delgado, G. (1993) *Multicultural issues in deafness*, White Plains, NY: Longman.

Comerford, D.G. et al (1995) 'The Bradford and Airedale baby hearing project. An assessment of the impact of screening on the earlier detection of infant hearing loss', *Clinical Otolaryngology*, vol 20, pp 536-9.

Cooper, J. (1995) 'Health needs assessment for children with hearing impairment', unpublished draft report, Bradford Health Authority.

Darr, A., Jones, L., Ahmad, W.I.U. and Nisar, G. (1997) *A directory of initiatives and services with minority ethnic deaf people*, Social Policy Research Unit, York University/Ethnicity and Social Policy Research Unit, University of Bradford.

Davis, A. et al (1997) 'A critical review of the role of neonatal hearing screening in the detection of congenital hearing impairment', *Health Technology Assessment*, vol 1, no 10.

Fletcher, L. (1987) *A language for Ben*, London: Souvenir Press.

Glendinning, C. (1985) *A single door*, London: Allen and Unwin.

Gregory, S. (1973) *The deaf child and his family*, London: George Allen and Unwin.

Gregory, S., Bishop, J. and Sheldon, L. (1995) *Deaf young people and their families*, Cambridge: Cambridge University Press.

Hall, D.M.B. (1991) *Health for all children*, Report of the Second Joint Working Party on Child Health Surveillance.

Health Education Authority (1997) *Many voices, one message: Guidance for the development and translation of health information*, London: Health Education Authority.

Hill, S.A. (1994) *Managing sickle cell disease in low income families*, Philadephia: Temple University Press.

Hopkins, A. and Bahl, V. (eds) (1993) *Access to health care for people from black and ethnic minorities*, London: Royal College of Physicians.

Jones, L. and Pullen, G. (1990) *Inside we are all equal. A social policy survey of deaf people in Europe*, London: ECRS.

Kurtz, Z. (1993) 'Better health for black and ethnic minority children and young people', in A. Hopkins and V. Bahl (eds) *Access to health care for people from black and ethnic minorities*, London: Royal College of Physicians.

Mahon, M., Wells, B. and Tarplee, C. (1995) *Conversational strategies of deaf children and their families where English is the second language*, Final Report to the ESRC.

Meherali, R. (1985) *The deaf Asian child and his family*, unpublished MA thesis, University of Nottingham, cited in Open University (1991) Unit 5, *Deaf people in hearing worlds*, Buckingham: Open University Press.

Meherali, R. (1994) 'Being black and deaf', in C. Laurenzi (ed) (1994) *Keep deaf children in mind: Current issues in mental health*, Leeds: National Deaf Children's Society.

Miles, M. (1993) 'Concepts of mental retardation in Pakistan: towards cross-cultural and historical perspectives', *Disability, Handicap and Society*, vol 7, pp 235-55.

Naeem, Z. and Newton, V. (1996) 'The prevalence of sensori-neural hearing loss in Asian children', *British Journal of Audiology*, vol 30, no 5, pp 332-40.

NDCS (National Deaf Children's Society) (1990) *Audiological services for children: Recommended practice in the UK*, London: NDCS.

NDCS (1994) *Quality standards in paediatric audiology: volume 1, Guidelines for the early identification of hearing impairment*, London: NDCS.

NDCS (1994) *Quality standards in paediatric audiology: volume II, The audiological management of the child: A consultation document*, London: NDCS.

Parsons, L., Macfarlane, A. and Golding, J. (1993) 'Pregnancy, birth and maternity care', in W.I.U. Ahmad (ed) *'Race' and health in contemporary Britain*, Buckingham: Open University Press.

Robinson, K. (1991) *The children of silence*, London: Gollancz.

Shackman, J. (1985) *The right to be understood*, Cambridge: National Extension College.

Sharma, A. and Love, D. (1991) *A change in approach: A report on the experience of deaf people from black and ethnic minority communities*, London: The Royal Association in Aid of Deaf People.

Sloper, T. and Turner, S. (1992) 'Service needs of families of children with severe physical disability', *Child: Care, Health and Development*, vol 18, pp 259-82.

SMAC (1994) *Report of the standing medical advisory committee on sickle cell, thalassaemia and other haemoglobinopathies*, London: DoH.

Smaje, C. (1994) *Health, 'race' and ethnicity: Making sense of the evidence*, London: King's Fund.

Social Services Inspectorate (1997) *Better management, better care: The Sixth Annual Report of the Chief Inspector*, London: HMSO.

Stuart, O. (1992) 'Race and disability: just a double oppression?', *Disability, Handicap and Society*, vol 7, no 2, pp 177-88.

Twigg, J. (1992) *Carers: Research and practice*, London: HMSO.

Twigg, J. and Atkin, K. (1994) *Carers perceived: Policy and practice in informal care*, Buckingham: Open University Press.

Warrier, S. (1988) 'Marriage, maternity and female economic activity: Gujerati mothers in Britain', in S. Westwood and P. Bhachu (eds) *Enterprising women: Ethnicity, economy and gender relations*, London: Routledge.

Watson, E. (1984) 'Health of infants and use of health services by mothers of different ethnic groups in East London', *Community Medicine*, vol 6, pp 127-35.

# Appendix A: Methods

In developing our research design, we had a number of considerations. Our primary interest was the perspectives of parents and of health professionals. However, within the health services, a range of professionals are involved with parents of deaf children depending on the particular stage in the diagnostic process or the child's age. Health service professionals often also work closely with the education service or other agencies. The design therefore had to be able to encompass the following:

- provide parents' accounts of their experiences, interaction with health services, social and family support, coping strategies, ideas about aetiology, views about language and communication, and types of services they find particularly helpful;
- provide practitioners' perspectives – such as health visitors, GPs, ENT surgeons, audiological physicians, audiological technicians – on service delivery to individual families as well as to Asian and non-Asian families more generally, their views on service organisation, interagency working, and means of improving services;
- assess interagency working between health and other services, especially education and social services;
- enable an assessment of how health commissioners establish priorities for purchasing services and how purchasing mechanisms may be used as a vehicle for improving healthcare for young deaf children.

The initial phase of research included a small number of informal interviews with parents of deaf children and practitioners from health, peripatetic education service and social services. These allowed us to gauge our understanding of the issues highlighted in the relevant literature and policy knowledge against what was regarded as significant by these respondents. A one-day workshop was also held, jointly, with a related project (Ahmad et al, 1998) where a number of minority ethnic, both voluntary and paid, workers with deaf people and their families discussed a range of issues related to access and service needs. The fieldwork consisted of two main stages. In stage one, we interviewed parents of deaf children under five years of age. In stage two, our focus was on providers in health, social and education services, and on health commissioners. Ethical approval was obtained from all the local ethics committees in the fieldwork localities. In addition, a research ethics statement was drafted and adhered to on the suggestion of the Project Advisory Committee.

## Stage one: interviews with parents

In total, interviews were conducted with 26 parents of deaf children; all except one were from Muslim families, the majority were of Pakistani origin. Only parents of children with long-term sensori-neural hearing loss, which ranged from 'upper half of moderate' to 'profound', were included. The profile of children, details of whether the interviews were conducted with the mother or the father, brief family profile including family history of deafness, age of diagnosis and degree of deafness, and language of interview is provided in Appendix B.

Apart from one child who was aged seven at the time of the interview, all the other children were aged five or under. Three children had other disabilities as well as deafness. Nine interviews were conducted with parents who had two or more deaf children. Two of the children had one deaf parent. Of the 26 interviews, 21 were conducted with mothers and five with fathers. Six of the interviews with mothers and one with a father were conducted in Punjabi or Urdu, the rest were conducted in English. Parents were given the choice to be interviewed by a same gender interviewer, and in the language of their choice. Aliya Darr, a female researcher on a related project (Darr et al, 1997; Ahmad et al, 1998), conducted 11 of the interviews with women, where the respondents had expressed a preference for a female interviewer.

Prior to the interview, respondents were sent a personalised letter (in English and Urdu) and an information sheet about the project and the interview (again in English and Urdu). Considering problems of literacy, we also sent the same information on an audio-tape in English, Urdu and Punjabi. In most cases, where the parents had a telephone, we made an appointment, over the telephone, to conduct the interview. Where they did not have a telephone, we arranged appointments through letters and/or made opportunistic visits during which a time for conducting the interview was agreed. Respondents were assured confidentiality. This was particularly important considering that we would also be interviewing healthcare and other service providers with whom they had contact.

A topic guide was used to structure the interviews. The topics of discussion included basic personal and demographic details; questions about first suspicions; immediate actions; the process of seeking help; contact with hospitals, the diagnosis and response to diagnosis;

information needs and sources; everyday life of the deaf child; family communication; language, culture and identity; and experience of services. Within each of these broad topics, specific prompts were used to aid discussion. All except one of the interviews were tape-recorded. Most interviews lasted about one hour. Parents spoke freely of their experiences without objecting to any of the topics under discussion. Some parents felt emotional about certain aspects of their experience but opted to continue the interview or returned to those sensitive experiences later in the interview.

As we wished to explore both service provision to individual families and the nature of interpersonal and interagency collaboration both in relation to these families and more generally, we therefore requested from parents names of two professionals to interview, one of whom was to be from the health service and the other from some other agency, whom the families had found useful.

## Stage two: interviews with practitioners

A range of practitioners including, within the health services, both primary healthcare and hospital-based practitioners, as well as the peripatetic education service, play an important role in identification of deafness and provision of support to deaf children and their families. The names of practitioners given by parents provided an important starting point for the sample selection for this stage. However, these names were augmented for three reasons. First, there were some obvious gaps in the range of professionals being identified; most of the practitioners suggested by parents were health visitors, ENT or audiological consultants, or peripatetic teachers; often several parents named the same individuals. Secondly, as these practitioners were concentrated in the same localities as the parents, we wished to include practitioners from other areas of West Yorkshire to gain a broader perspective on the organisation of services. Thirdly, we had to augment the sample with health commissioners who would generally not be known to parents. Therefore, in addition to the names suggested by parents, we selected other professionals through purposive, snowball sampling. In doing so we attempted to have a spread of different professions and people from different localities within West Yorkshire, although with a bias in favour of the localities where parents were interviewed.

As with parents, professionals were sent information about the project along with the request for an interview. On the basis of a preliminary analysis of the interviews with parents, and further discussions with service professionals, a topic guide was developed for interviews with professionals. The topics included: background information about the respondent; role and scope of the service; mixed economy of care; interprofessional and interagency collaboration and service coordination; diagnosis; views on aetiology; cochlear implants and hearing aids; services for Asian deaf children and their families; ideas about deafness, culture and identity; and their views about the shape of an 'ideal' service. This topic guide, however, needed to be customised to take account of what parents had said about certain practitioners or services. Questions about specific families were couched in terms of generalities to ensure confidentiality. The guides also had to take into account the roles of different professionals. Although there may be much overlap between what may be appropriate to discuss with a health commissioner and a peripatetic teacher, there was clearly the need to consider their different responsibilities and interests. As with the parents, confidentiality was assured to all respondents. Most interviews lasted about one hour; all were tape-recorded.

The final sample consisted of 44 respondents made up of:

- 18 providers from the health service, including health visitors, ENT surgeons, community paediatricians, senior clinical medical officers, paediatric audiological technicians, managers, and people working in the genetics service;
- 14 practitioners from the peripatetic education service, many of whom worked closely with the local hospitals and were involved in supporting and advising parents following diagnosis;
- 6 practitioners from social services;
- 6 health commissioners.

## Analysis

All interviews were tape-recorded and fully transcribed. Interviews which were conducted in Punjabi or Urdu went through an interim stage of verbatim interpretation into English onto another audio-tape, before being transcribed. The interpretation was done by the researchers.

In analysing transcripts we were interested in reconstructing the key themes from the parents' and professionals' accounts. For reasons of comparison an attempt was made to, where possible, use similar analytic categories for analysis of the two stages of fieldwork. The topic guides provided the starting point for coding categories. These categories were further expanded and modified through detailed analysis of the transcripts.

## Confidentiality

We have taken care to maintain confidentiality of our respondents. The names in the family profile (Appendix B) have been changed and the localities have not been identified. However, as the job titles for some of the professionals are idiosyncratic to certain localities, and in the case of some specialities, there are very few such people in West Yorkshire, we have not offered a pen portrait of professionals interviewed. Where appropriate in the text of the report, and where we can be sure that the respondent will not be easily identified, we have given them generic job titles.

# Appendix B: Profile of families

The following list provides a brief profile of families and children involved in the research study. To preserve anonymity we have changed their names.

Jamal is seven years old. He has one older and three younger siblings, all hearing. Jamal was diagnosed at the age of three years and six months. The interview was conducted with his mother in Punjabi/Urdu.

Naila, aged two, is profoundly deaf. She has a younger brother aged four months. Naila was diagnosed around the age of one year and two months. The interview was conducted with her mother in Punjabi/Urdu.

Marya is four years and six months old. She is profoundly deaf. She has an older brother who is hearing, an older sister and a younger sister both profoundly deaf, and another younger brother aged three who is hearing. Marya was diagnosed at age two months. The interview was conducted with the mother in Punjabi/Urdu.

Naseer is two years and two months old and is severely deaf. He has an older brother who is disabled and deaf, and two other brothers who are hearing. The interview was conducted with the mother in Punjabi/Urdu.

Amjad is two years old. He has moderate to severe deafness with permanent conductive hearing loss. Amjad has three other siblings who are all older and hearing. The interview was conducted with his mother in Punjabi/Urdu.

Faisal is one year and nine months old and profoundly deaf. He has a step sister who is hearing and also has deaf cousins. Faisal's mother and father were interviewed separately in English.

Jabbar is three years old. Jabbar has moderate to severe deafness and also has other disabilities. He has a hearing older brother. The interview was conducted with the father, in English.

Laila is aged one year and nine months and is profoundly deaf. She has a younger hearing brother. She was diagnosed at just over one year of age. The interview was conducted with her father, in English.

Khalid is two years and nine months old. He is profoundly deaf and has a younger hearing brother. The interview was conducted with the mother, in English.

Omar is four years old. His deafness is regarded to be in the upper half of moderate. He has a deaf older brother. Omar was diagnosed at nearly two years of age. The interview was conducted with the mother, in English.

Khalil is five years old with moderate to severe deafness. He has a younger sister who is also moderately deaf. Khalil was diagnosed at the age of four years. The interview was conducted with the mother, in English.

Rashid is two years old and is moderately deaf. He has a older hearing sibling. The interview was conducted with the mother, in English.

Sahera is one year and six months old and is severely deaf. She has a younger baby sister whose hearing is yet to be assessed. Sahera has four deaf cousins. The interview was conducted with the mother, in English.

Humaira is 18 months old and is the youngest of three children. She is severely deaf and disabled. Humaira has an older deaf brother with the same disability and a hearing sister. She was diagnosed as deaf at three months and her older brother was diagnosed at three years and six months of age. The interview was conducted with the mother, in English.

Charles is two years and two weeks old. His parents did not think that he was deaf although a diagnosis was made at around the age of one year. He has four older siblings, all hearing. The interview was conducted with both parents, in English.

Adeeba is five years old. She has a hearing younger brother, aged one year and six months. The interview was conducted with her mother, in English.

Nasreen is two years and nine months old and is profoundly deaf. She has a hearing older brother. The interview was conducted with the mother, in Punjabi. Nasreen has developed good speech for her age.

Qadeer is six years old and is partially deaf. He has four older sisters who are hearing and a younger sister aged two years and six months who is awaiting hearing assessment. The interview was conducted with his father, in Punjabi/Urdu.

Rabia is five years old. She is severely deaf and also has sight problems. Her older sister is moderately deaf and she has two hearing siblings. One of the parents is partially deaf and there are other deaf people in the family. Rabia's eldest sister was diagnosed at the age of six years. The interview was conducted with the mother, in English.

Shahid is five years old and is severely deaf. He has an older brother and a sister, who are hearing. The interview was conducted with Shahid's mother, in Punjabi/Urdu.

Zahida is three years and six months old and her deafness is assessed as upper half of moderate. Zahida has an older brother, who is hearing. The interview was conducted with the mother, in English.

Najma is six years of age and is profoundly deaf. Najma has two younger sisters who are also profoundly deaf. She was diagnosed at the age of six months. Najma's father is also profoundly deaf. The interview was conducted with the mother, in Punjabi/Urdu.

Tahera is two years and six months old. She is profoundly deaf and was diagnosed at age one year and six months. Tahera has no siblings. The interview was conducted with her mother, in English.

Haleema is two years and six months old and was diagnosed as profoundly deaf at one and a half years. Haleema does not have any siblings. The interview was conducted with Haleema's mother in English.

Taslim is five years old, an only child and profoundly deaf. The interview was conducted with his mother, in Purijabi/Urdu.